To people at risk of and with diabetes:
May the words on the pages of this book encourage you to take
actions now to eat healthfully day after day. May healthier eating
help you become and stay healthier for years to come.

Table of Contents

Section **One** Diabetes, Nutrition,
and Healthy Eating Basics

Section Two Foods by Group

Section Three Putting Healthy Eating into Action

Introduction to 4th Edition

By opening the pages of this book you have signaled that you are ready to learn how to eat healthier. Great! You may have been diagnosed with diabetes yesterday, have had diabetes for many years, have just been told you are at high risk for developing type 2 diabetes, or are concerned about a family member or friend with diabetes. Whatever your situation, this book will help you uncover the details about healthy eating with diabetes—from the basics of what to eat, to the practical skills of shopping, planning healthy meals, and even eating healthy restaurant meals.

Hands down, healthy eating day after day is the most difficult and challenging part of taking care of diabetes, especially today in our fast-paced convenience-driven world. *Diabetes Meal Planning Made Easy* helps you learn which changes to make in your eating habits and food choices. This book provides you with lots of easy ways to make these changes. It also helps you analyze your current food habits and lifestyle to determine your helpful and harmful habits. It will also help you continue to enjoy the many foods you love to eat. Yes, that's right, you don't have to give up the foods you enjoy!

A healthy eating plan is an essential component of your diabetes care—whether or not you take blood-glucose-lowering medications or other medications to control your blood pressure, lipids, and more. As you thumb through the pages ahead, keep in mind that today, research suggests that the best way to stay healthy with diabetes over the years is to get and keep your blood glucose, blood lipids, and blood pressure in your target ranges—you'll soon know these as your diabetes ABCs.

If you have opened this book to find a one-size-fits-all diet or a magic bullet approach to weight loss, you've come to the *wrong* place. (Weight loss and diabetes control take persistence and hard work and you'll get plenty of tips for success in the pages ahead.) You've come to the right place if you want an approach to help you slowly change your eating habits for the rest of your life, lose weight (if you need to), and keep the weight off.

If you are at high risk for type 2 diabetes or already have type 2 diabetes, it's highly likely that some weight loss will benefit your health. Keeping the weight off will be just as important. Every chapter is chock full of tips and strategies for healthier eating as well as weight loss and long-term control.

Your goal should be to develop a healthy eating plan that you are willing and able to follow the rest of your life. That's how long you'll have diabetes.

Diabetes Meal Planning Made Easy is divided into three sections:

Section 1: Diabetes, Nutrition, and Healthy Eating Basics

Learn about nutrition basics, including carbohydrate, protein, and fat. Review the healthy eating guidelines that are beneficial for everyone, from young to old, as well as specific recommendations for people with various types of diabetes. Also learn about vitamins, minerals, and supplements and find out how much sodium to include in your eating plan.

Section 2: Foods by Group

Learn about the food groups. These include the starches and grains, fruits and fruit juices, vegetables (non-starchy), meats, and dairy foods.

You'll also find out about other kinds of food you eat: fats and oils, sugar and sweets, alcoholic and non-alcoholic beverages, and even mixed-up foods like pizza, soups, and frozen meals. Learn which nutrients are provided by the foods in each food group and discover easy ways to eat more or less of those foods to achieve your diabetes goals. You'll also read the stories of how people with diabetes, like you, have been able to set and achieve their healthy eating and diabetes goals.

Section 3: Putting Healthy Eating into Action

This section helps you apply the knowledge and strategies you've learned in the first two sections to plan healthy meals and snacks every day. Learn how to set short-term goals and evaluate their success to achieve and maintain healthy behavior changes, practice portion control, read food and Nutrition Facts labels, and eat healthier restaurant meals.

Think of your healthy eating plan and healthier habits as long-term works in progress. Don't try to change everything at once. Take one step at a time. Keep in mind that any change you make to eat healthier is a step in the right direction. Also, keep in mind that none of this is easy. Think about finding a supportive network to maximize your success. Local support groups, Weight Watchers meetings, or online diabetes and/or weight control support networks are a great place to start.

Keep in mind that success breeds success. Once you are successful at making one change, you're likely to be more successful at making the next change and the one after that. Making changes will become easier for you as time goes on. This is true whether you are trying to make healthier food choices or be more physically active— another important part of staying healthy with diabetes.

Before you read on, spend a few minutes jotting down some notes about your eating habits. Create a form like the one on the next page. If you are honest with yourself, you can learn a lot about your current food choices and eating habits. Next, it's time to start changing your habits for good, one step at a time.

TIME	FOOD	FOOD PREPARATION	AMOUNT YOU EAT

The pages ahead contain everything you need to know about healthy eating with diabetes. Don't worry about what you've eaten and how you've lived in the past. Start changing your eating habits now to get and keep your blood glucose, blood lipids, and blood pressure on target. These goals are your key to staying healthy with diabetes. Don't delay; jump in!

SECTION ONE

Diabetes, Nutrition, and Healthy Eating Basics

Chapter 1

A Few Bits and Bites about Diabetes

What You'll Learn:

- what diabetes is and how it affects your body and why you'll want to track your levels over time
- the target goals for blood glucose, blood lipids, and blood pressure—your ABCs
- how pre-diabetes (being at high risk for type 2) can progress to type 2 diabetes and what you can do to slow down this process
- the benefits of weight loss and physical activity to your short- and long-term health

What Is Diabetes?

Before you dig in to learn about healthier eating, take a few minutes to learn more about diabetes and what you can do to slow down the progress of this disease. If you have diabetes, your body has difficulty converting the food you eat into energy you can use.

After you eat, your body breaks down some of the food into glucose, or sugar, which is the basic fuel for all the cells in your body. Insulin, a hormone produced by the beta cells in the pancreas, helps take the glucose from your blood to the cells. When you have pre-diabetes or type 2 diabetes, two things are going wrong with this process. First, your body is unable to keep up with the demand for large amounts of insulin. Very often this is because you are carrying around excess weight. Second, because your body has become resistant to the insulin your pancreas does make, you are not able to efficiently use the insulin you make. You have both insufficient insulin production and insulin resistance— key features of pre-diabetes and type 2 diabetes. The result is that glucose builds up in your blood, instead of getting into your cells via insulin to be used for energy. Over the years, high blood glucose levels can damage your kidneys, eyes, and nerves.

Managing your diabetes means working to keep your blood glucose levels as close to normal as possible. Unfortunately, people with diabetes, and particularly type 2 diabetes, also often have high blood pressure and unhealthy blood lipid levels: HDL (good) cholesterol is too low, triglycerides are too high, and LDL (bad) cholesterol is too high. These problems are caused by excessive weight and insulin resistance.

It's the combination of high blood glucose levels, high blood pressure, and abnormal lipid levels that can cause the more serious complications of diabetes, including heart and blood vessel diseases. People with diabetes are six times more likely to have a heart attack and four times more like to have a stroke than people without diabetes. Heart and blood vessel diseases are the leading causes of medical problems and death for people with diabetes. Enough bad news, the good news is that just a small amount of weight loss can improve all of these problems.

Many people need to take medications to manage blood glucose, blood pressure, and abnormal lipids to stay on target. Achieving these ABC goals can help keep you healthy for years to come.

Know Your ABCs

The three targets of effective diabetes management are known as the ABCs:

Target ABC Goals		
A is for...	**B** is for...	**C** is for...
A1C or blood glucose	Blood pressure	Cholesterol or blood lipids
ADA Recommendation	ADA Recommendation	ADA Recommendation
A1C: <7%	<130/80 mmHg	LDL: <100 mg/dl
Fasting and before meals blood glucose: 70–130 mg/dl		HDL: >40 mg/dl (men) >50 mg/dl (women)
Blood glucose 2 hours after the start of a meal: <180 mg/dl		Triglycerides: <150 mg/dl

The American Diabetes Association recommends ABC goals for people with diabetes. Your health care provider can help you decide which goals are right for you.

Pre-diabetes (High Risk) and Type 2 Diabetes

About 57 million people in the United States have "pre-diabetes," a condition in which blood glucose levels are higher than normal but not high enough to be diagnosed as diabetes. (Pre-diabetes can also be considered being at high risk for diabetes.)

In the last decade, research has given health care providers a better understanding of how pre-diabetes can progress into type 2 diabetes if left untreated. Read about how pre-diabetes and type 2 can happen and how you can prevent or delay it if you are at high risk (see Progression from Normal Blood Glucose to Pre-Diabetes and Type 2 chart, page 7).

Here's what happens progressively:
- *Excess weight and inactivity initiate the problem.* Excess adipose tissue (fat) releases markers of chronic inflammation into the bloodstream.
- *Inflammation causes insulin resistance to escalate.* Inflammation inhibits the action of insulin made in the pancreas, so your body is not able to use your insulin effectively, and also has a greater demand for it. This can damage your body's tissues, yet you will likely be unaware that it is happening.
- *With inflammation and insulin resistance the body powers up the beta cells to put out more insulin.* Larger amounts of insulin are put out into the bloodstream to work on keeping blood glucose normal. This is when blood pressure starts to rise and blood lipids become abnormal.
- *Insulin production from beta cells begins to dwindle.* Blood glucose levels slowly start to rise above normal. Initially, blood glucose levels after meals tend to be higher before fasting levels.
- *Blood glucose climbs slowly.* The beta cells slowly become exhausted and can't make enough insulin to keep blood glucose at normal levels. This is when blood glucose levels rise and the A1C level rises high enough to put you at high risk for diabetes. This subtle process can take 10 years or more for adults. Research shows it may happen more quickly in children and adolescents.
- *The pancreas can no longer keep up with the body's demand for insulin.* The blood glucose rises to levels that are diagnostic for diabetes. Interestingly, at diagnosis people have already lost between 50 and 80% of their beta cells. At this point many people usually need to start taking a blood glucose–lowering medication, often metformin.

● *Over time the ability to make insulin continues to dwindle and insulin resistance continues.* To keep blood glucose levels in target ranges, you'll need to progress your blood glucose–lowering medication. Eventually, many people who live long enough with type 2 will need to take insulin by injection.

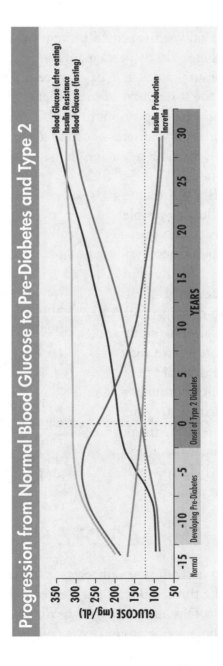

Progression from Normal Blood Glucose to Pre-Diabetes and Type 2

Pre-diabetes (High Risk of Type 2 Diabetes): What You Can Do?

A large study started in the late 1990s called the Diabetes Prevention Program (DPP) showed that people at risk for type 2 diabetes who lost a small amount of weight (5–7% or about 10–20 pounds) and became more physically active, could prevent or delay the development of type 2 diabetes. Study participants were active for 150 minutes a week (30 minutes a day, five days a week). People lost weight and kept it off for the three years of the initial study by eating fewer calories, less fat, and smaller portions of food. The participants experienced other benefits of weight loss, such as lowered blood pressure, improved blood lipids, and a reduction in medicines needed to control these conditions.

The DPPOS (Outcome Study), which is following people in the DPP, shows that it's best to focus on keeping off these few pounds by eating healthy and being physically active. Losing weight and keeping weight off is challenging enough. This study showed that support—from diabetes educators, health care providers, a weight control group, or friends—can be critical to your success. For this reason, think about finding a local or online support network to help you with your efforts long term.

> ● **QUICK TIP**
>
> Key medical benefits from weight loss happen with the first 10 to 15 pounds you lose. There is no need to get down to an unrealistically low weight to enjoy these benefits. The key is to keep this small amount of weight off for good.

A Diagnosis of Type 2 Diabetes

You may be diagnosed with type 2 diabetes just after your blood glucose level crosses the threshold, or it may be years before you discover that your blood glucose is high enough to be diagnosed as diabetes. In addition, you may be carrying around extra pounds. These factors and

Blood Glucose Levels in Pre-diabetes and Diabetes

	Normal	Pre-diabetes*	Diabetes**
Fasting	<100 mg/dl	100–125 mg/dl	≥126 mg/dl
2 hours after eating		<140 mg/dl	≥140–200 mg/dl 200 mg/dl
Anytime			Diabetes symptoms plus casual glucose ≥200 mg/dl

*People with pre-diabetes or early-onset type 2 diabetes may have a normal fasting plasma glucose level but a higher than normal level 2 hours after eating.

**A diagnosis of diabetes must be confirmed on a subsequent day by measuring fasting blood glucose, blood glucose levels 2 hours after eating, or casual (anytime) blood glucose.

others will influence how you and your health care provider will treat your diabetes.

Keep in mind that the care of type 2 diabetes has changed a great deal over the past few years. That's because more has been learned about the progressive changes noted above. Recent research indicates that you can slow down the progression of type 2 diabetes—and reduce the chances of heart and blood vessel complications—by keeping your glucose levels on target day to day and year to year. For this reason current ADA recommendations suggest that you start taking one of several blood glucose–lowering medications as soon as you are diagnosed with type 2 diabetes. This doesn't negate the importance of losing some weight and becoming more physically active. These actions can help increase your insulin sensitivity and, along with the medication, improve your ABCs.

If your health care provider suggests blood glucose–lowering medication, don't fight it. Normal or near-normal blood glucose levels will help keep you healthy. As time goes on, don't fight taking more medication or adding a new one to keep your blood glucose under control (see Know Your ABCs, page 5). If your health care provider suggests taking insulin to achieve glucose control, try not to fight this or put it off for too long. With thinner, sharper needles, convenient pens or pumps, and newer insulins, taking insulin is easier than ever before.

Key Features of a Diabetes Treatment Plan

Regardless of the medications you use over the years to manage your glucose levels, blood lipids, and blood pressure, research shows that there are three other key features for a solid treatment plan for diabetes. These are:

- healthy eating
- achieving and maintaining a healthy weight
- being physically active.

You can start to take charge of your plan by reading this book and deciding which changes you can make to live a healthier life with diabetes.

The Nutrients Big and Small

What You'll Learn:

- a definition of calories and how your body uses them
- what the big nutrients are—carbohydrate, protein, and fats
- what the small nutrients are—vitamins, minerals, and water

As you set out to learn about healthy eating with diabetes and the ins and outs of meal planning, you'll need to learn a few nutrition basics. Familiarity with these basic nutrition terms will help you understand your diabetes nutrition goals as well as how this book breaks foods into food groups.

Calories

Food supplies energy in the form of calories (units of energy), and the body uses calories to function and to move. Your body's need for calories, or energy, never stops, even when you sleep. The number of calories you need each day depends on many factors. For starters, these factors include your sex, your size, what you do during the day, and how physically active you are outside of your daily activities.

The calories in foods come from one of three macro—or big—nutrients. These are carbohydrate, protein, and fat. A fourth source of calories is alcohol.

Your body needs insulin to be able to put the calories you eat to work. Insulin is a hormone that is made in and secreted from the beta cells of the pancreas. If you have diabetes, your body has trouble supplying insulin to your cells. With type 1 diabetes, your body is no longer able to make any insulin. In type 2 diabetes, your body may not make enough insulin to manage your blood glucose (insulin deficiency) and/or may not effectively use the insulin made in the pancreas (insulin resistance). Both situations make it harder to manage blood glucose levels.

● **QUICK TIP**

Think of foods as "packages" of varying amounts of carbohydrate, protein, and fat. For example, a slice of bread contains mostly carbohydrate with a small amount of protein. A piece of turkey contains mainly protein with a small amount of fat.

The Big Nutrients

Carbohydrates

Carbohydrates are the main source of calories that provide your body with energy. They are your body's preferred source of energy, because they provide energy in a form that's easy for your body to break down and use. After you eat, your body breaks down carbohydrate into glucose that travels to your blood stream. To help the cells use this glucose, the body normally releases insulin from the pancreas.

Carbohydrates fall into three general categories: sugars, starches, and fibers. Carbohydrates contain 4 calories of energy per gram. They are the main source of energy that raises your blood glucose levels.

Carbohydrate Sources

These foods contain most of their calories from carbohydrate:

- starches, such as breads, cereals, pasta, and starchy vegetables
- sugars, such as regular soda, gum drops, and syrups
- sweets, such as desserts, ice cream, and candy
- vegetables (nonstarchy), such as lettuce, broccoli, and carrots
- fruits, such as apples, oranges, fruit juices, and raisins
- dairy foods, such as milk and yogurt (cheese contains just a small amount of carbohydrate)

Proteins

Proteins are a source of calories from foods that provide energy, but unlike carbohydrates, they aren't your body's preferred source of energy. Proteins are made up of chains of amino acids—the building blocks of protein. Different sequences of amino acids create different proteins. Once you eat protein, the body breaks it down into amino

Protein Sources

These foods contain most of their calories from protein:

- red meats (beef, lamb, pork, and veal)
- poultry (chicken, turkey), seafood, fish, and shellfish
- cheese
- eggs

These foods contain moderate amounts of their calories from protein:

- dairy foods, milk, and yogurt
- legumes, beans, and peas
- nuts

These foods contain small amounts of their calories from protein:

- starches, such as breads, cereals, pasta, and starchy vegetables
- vegetables (nonstarchy), such as lettuce, broccoli, and carrots
- fruits, such as apples, oranges, fruit juice, and raisins

acids, which are used to build, repair, and maintain the body's tissues. Protein contains 4 calories of energy per gram.

Fats

Fats are a source of calories from foods that provide energy, but they aren't your body's preferred source of energy. Calories from fat are used for energy if the body doesn't have enough calories from carbohydrate. Insulin plays a role in helping your body store fat in your cells.

Fat provides a concentrated source of calories at 9 per gram. That's more than double the calories per gram for carbohydrate and protein. There are four different types of fats—saturated, trans, polyunsaturated, and monounsaturated. Fat-containing foods have varying amounts of these fats. Some of the fat you eat is in the food itself, like the fat in meat, chicken, and cheese. Some fat is added to foods, such as margarine on a potato, cream cheese on a bagel, dressing on a salad, or the fat from oil used in frying.

Fat Sources

These foods contain nearly all of their calories from fat:

- oils (all types)
- margarine, butter, and cream cheese
- salad dressings, mayonnaise, and sour cream

These foods contain many of their calories from fat:

- nuts and seeds
- sausage and bacon (regular)

These foods contain varying amounts of their calories from fat, depending on several factors, such as the cut of meat, whether the poultry is eaten with skin on or off, and whether the food is regular, low-fat, or fat-free:

- red meats (beef, lamb, pork, and veal)
- poultry
- seafood, fish, and shellfish
- cheese
- eggs
- milk and yogurt

Alcohol

Alcohol is obviously not a nutrient that the body needs to function, but many people choose to include alcohol in their eating plan. It is important to understand that alcohol contains 7 calories of energy per gram. It falls midway between the calories of energy per gram of carbohydrate and protein at 4 and fat at 9. Clearly, the calories from alcohol can add up. Another downside of alcohol is that the hefty dose of calories provides no nutritional value. You'll learn more about the use of alcohol with diabetes in chapter 17.

● QUICK TIP

Try to limit your consumption of alcohol to one drink per day for women and two drinks per day for men.

The Small Nutrients

Vitamins and Minerals

Vitamins and minerals provide no calories. They are contained within foods and are essential for the body to function properly. They help your body use the food you eat to make your body function. Each vitamin and mineral that your body needs performs a unique task to keep your body working and keep you healthy. In fact, beyond the known vitamins and minerals that foods offer, there are also hundreds of naturally occurring substances in foods that may protect against chronic health problems.

A key message about healthy eating in this book is to look to food first to get most of your essential nutrients. In the pages ahead, you'll learn more about the importance of eating a wide variety of foods to get all the vitamins and minerals you need. Learn more about vitamins, minerals, and dietary supplements in chapter 7.

Water

Water makes up about 60% of your body weight. Water is considered an essential nutrient, and a constant supply of water is vital to the proper functioning of your body. Water contains no calories. You get water from the liquids you drink and the food you eat. Foods like vegetables, fruit, and milk contain a high percentage of water. People need about 8 cups (64 ounces) of fluids per day. This varies greatly with the climate you live in, the type of work you do, and your level of physical activity. It's important to keep yourself properly hydrated and to use thirst as an indicator of

● **QUICK TIP**

Water makes up 60% of your body weight. Make sure you drink at least 8 glasses (64 ounces) of fluids per day.

how much water or other liquids you need. By far, water is the best beverage to choose to quench your thirst. You can learn more about choosing healthy beverages in chapter 16.

The next two chapters describe the general healthy eating guide-lines and the specific diabetes nutrition recommendations. This information will help you put the nutrition puzzle together.

Chapter

Healthy Eating Guidelines for All

What You'll Learn:

- the nine key healthy eating guidelines for everyone
- what and how people typically eat
- how the healthy eating guidelines for everyone match the healthy eating goals for people with diabetes

As a person with diabetes, do you wonder whether you should follow the healthy eating guidelines for everyone or if you need to follow a special set of guidelines? Do you wonder if you can (or should) lean toward vegetarianism or continue being a vegetarian if you already are? If you have heart problems, do you wonder whether you need to integrate yet another set of recommendations? Facing all these questions can be confusing, but don't despair! Take a deep breath and get ready for a lot of good news and easy-to-follow healthy eating guidelines.

Today, most nutrition advice is quite simple and straightforward. In this chapter, you'll see that the healthy eating guidelines suggested for everyone are very much in sync with the nutrition recommendations from the American Diabetes Association (ADA), which you'll get the full details about in chapter 4. In fact, these guidelines are in sync with healthy eating recommendations from other important health associations, like the American Heart Association and the American Cancer Society. In other words, when it comes to healthy eating guidelines, today there's essentially one set of guidelines for all.

Key Messages of the Dietary Guidelines

The Dietary Guidelines for Americans are revised every five years. The 2010 edition will be available late in 2010. Look for these on the United States Department of Agriculture's website, www.usda.gov. It's likely that nine key healthy eating messages will again emerge. Once you have read chapter 4, along with the rest of this book, you will see how closely these healthy eating guidelines echo the ADA recommendations.

1. **Eat a variety of foods within the basic food groups while you stay within your calorie needs. In other words, make your calories count.** Choose foods packed with vitamins and minerals. Don't use your calories on foods that are high in added fats and sugars. These foods end up being high in calories and low in nutrition.

2. **Control the amount of calories you eat to get to or stay at a healthy body weight.** Staying at a healthy body weight throughout your life is a key to good health. It helps you prevent or delay many diseases, such as type 2 diabetes, heart disease, and high blood pressure. To achieve and maintain a healthy body weight, don't eat more calories than you burn each day. If you find that your weight is creeping up, or has crept up over the years, shave off calories here and there by choosing healthier foods and burning more calories with physical activity.

3. **Increase the amount of fruits, vegetables, whole grains, and fat-free or low-fat milk and milk products you eat each day.** These foods provide essential vitamins and minerals to keep your body functioning properly. The best way to get the vitamins and minerals you need is to choose more of these healthy low-fat foods and less of the foods with lots of added fats and sugars.

4. **Choose fats wisely for good health.** Keep the amount of saturated fat and trans fats you eat as low as possible. Use healthier fats and oils—those that contain mainly polyunsaturated and monounsaturated fats.

5. **Choose carbohydrates wisely for good health.** Get about half the calories you eat each day from foods that contain healthy carbohydrates—whole grains, fruits, vegetables, and low-fat dairy foods. Choose fewer processed foods and foods with added sugars and fat.

6. **Choose and prepare foods with little salt.** Limit your sodium intake to no more than 2,300 milligrams a day or less. Research shows that it would be better to get sodium intake down to less than 1,500 milligrams a day, which is a challenge. Eat fewer processed and prepared foods and limit the amount of salt you add while preparing and eating food.

7. **If you drink alcoholic beverages, do so in moderation.** In other words, if you drink, don't drink too much and don't drink too much at one time. The recommendation is no more than 1 drink per day for women and 2 drinks per day for men.

8. **Keep food safe to eat.** Although this guideline doesn't directly have to do with nutrition, it's important to handle your food carefully to stay healthy. Practicing good hygiene is the watchword of food safety. Wash your hands regularly, and keep all surfaces that food touches clean. Wash all fruits and vegetables. Keep raw meats, poultry, and seafood away from cooked food. A surprising recommendation is that you don't need to wash or rinse meat or poultry. This prevents spreading potentially dangerous bacteria.

9. **Be physically active every day.** In late 2008, a new set of physical activity guidelines were published by the U.S. government giving recommendations for children, adults, and older adults. See daily activity recommendations on page 23. This report notes:
    1. some activity is better than none,
    2. activity is safe for almost everyone,
    3. health benefits of physical activity far outweigh the risk,
    4. people without a diagnosed condition and without symptoms of a medical problem do not need to discuss whether it is ok to be active with their health care provider.

Are your food habits similar to those of most people? Use the chart on the following pages to find out, and then decide which food choices and habits you may need to change.

Do you see a few themes here?
- Eat more fruits, vegetables, low-fat dairy foods, lean meats, and healthier fats and oils.
- Limit unhealthy saturated and trans fats.
- Limit foods that contain added fats (particularly saturated and trans fats) and added sugars.
- Choose minimally processed foods as much as possible.

These ideas may sound simple and repetitive of what you know, but following these guidelines regularly is easier said than done in today's world. Eating healthy takes determination and slow and steady behavior changes.

Recommendations for Daily Activity

Here are the basic recommendations:

Children and adolescents (6–17 years old): 1 hour (60 minutes) or more of moderate- or vigorous-intensity aerobic physical activity every day. They also should do muscle-strengthening and bone-strengthening activity at least 3 days per week.

Adults (aged 18–64 years old): 2 hours and 30 minutes a week of moderate-intensity, or 1 hour and 15 minutes (75 minutes) a week of vigorous-intensity aerobic physical activity, or an equivalent combination of moderate- and vigorous-intensity aerobic physical activity. Aerobic activity should be performed in episodes of at least 10 minutes, preferably spread throughout the week. Adults should also do muscle-strengthening activities that involve all major muscle groups performed on 2 or more days per week.

Older adults (aged 65 and older): Follow the guidelines for adults. If not possible, be as physically active as abilities allow. Avoid inactivity. Do exercises that maintain or improve balance to prevent falls.

To maintain a lower body weight after weight loss: Experts now agree that people who are trying to maintain weight loss will need to get about 60 minutes of moderate or 30 minutes of vigorous activity daily to prevent weight regain. Being physically active has been shown to be even more important to maintain weight loss than to lose weight.

Learn more at: http://www.cdc.gov/physicalactivity/every one/guidelines/index.html or http://www.health.gov/paguide lines/factsheetprof.aspx.

How We Eat Now—and How We Should Eat

Big and Small Nutrients	How We Eat	Dietary Guidelines*
Calories	Two-thirds of American adults are overweight. About 10–15% of children and adolescents are overweight. Many people consume too many calories to stay at a healthy weight. Men, on average, eat 2,500 calories a day. Women, on average, eat 1,800 calories a day. For many adults who get little physical activity, these calories are too high.	Many Americans need to lower the number of calories they eat each day to get to and stay at a healthier body weight.
Carbohydrates (Includes sugars, starches, whole grains, and dietary fiber.)	Americans eat about half their calories from carbohydrate, which is within the recommended range. The problem is not the quantity but the quality of carbohydrate. Americans eat: • too much added sugar from sugary drinks, desserts, and candy. • too few servings of whole grains, beans and peas, fruits, and green leafy and orange vegetables. • too little dairy food (about half the amount needed for calcium and other nutrients). • too little dietary fiber (about 10–14 grams/day).	Eat 45–65% of calories from carbohydrate. Do not eat more than 25% of calories from added sugars. Eat more dietary fiber. Choose more whole grains, fruits, vegetables, and low-fat dairy foods to achieve nutrition goals. Choose fewer foods and beverages with high amounts of added sugars.

How We Eat Now—and How We Should Eat
(continued)

Big and Small Nutrients	How We Eat	Dietary Guidelines*
Protein (Includes meats and nonmeat sources, such as cheese, eggs, and legumes.)	Americans eat more protein than necessary for good health. Americans also choose meats and other protein-dense foods that are too high in fat and unhealthy saturated fat. Americans do not choose enough of these sources of protein: • beans and peas • whole grains • low-fat dairy foods • fruits and vegetables.	You can eat 10–35% of calories from protein, but most people should aim for 15–25%. People with diabetes-related kidney disease should limit protein intake to 10–15%. Select lean cuts of meat, prepare foods in healthy ways, and eat smaller amounts of these foods. Choose healthier sources of protein, such as those in the list on the left.
Fats (Includes oils, shortening, salad dressings, meats, poultry, cheese, etc. Fats and foods that provide fat contain varying amounts of different fats and cholesterol.)	Americans eat about the right amount of calories from fat—in the range of 30–35%. But Americans eat: • too much saturated fat, at about 11% of calories. The main sources of saturated fat are cheese, beef, and milk. • too much trans fat, at about 3% of calories. About 80% of trans fat is from processed foods and 20% is from animal sources of food.	Eat 20–35% of calories as fat. Eat less saturated fat and as little trans fat as possible. Keep cholesterol under 200 mg/day. To accomplish these goals: • eat less full-fat cheese and fewer meats. • eat more fish and fatty fish. • choose low-fat or fat-free dairy foods.

(continues)

How We Eat Now—and How We Should Eat
(continued)

Big and Small Nutrients	How We Eat	Dietary Guidelines*
	• too much dietary cholesterol. Cholesterol intake is excessive for some men, but many people do not consume over 300 mg/day.	• choose healthy liquid vegetable oils, such as soybean, corn, canola, safflower, or olive oil. • eat small amounts of nuts.
Vitamins	Americans don't eat enough vitamins A, C, D, and E.	Eat more dairy foods, fruits, vegetables, whole grains, and healthy fats.
Minerals	Americans don't get enough calcium, potassium, and magnesium.	Eat more dairy foods, fruits, vegetables, and whole grains. Getting enough potassium can combat the effects of a high sodium intake.
Sodium	Americans eat too much sodium, an average of over 4,000 mg/day. Of that amount: • 75% is from processed foods. • 10% is natural salt in foods. • 5–10% is salt added at the table.	Consume no more than 2,300 mg/day. If you have high blood pressure, strive for no more than 1,500 mg/day and get enough potassium.
Alcohol	Most Americans drink alcohol.	Drink alcohol in moderation. Alcohol has both positive and negative health effects.

*These guidelines are based on the Dietary Reference Intakes from the Institute of Medicine of the National Academy of Sciences. They are acceptable ranges for adults and children other than infants and younger children.

Chapter 4

Healthy Eating Guidelines for Diabetes

What You'll Learn:

- the key principles of healthy eating with diabetes
- the goals of medical nutrition therapy (MNT), also known as nutrition counseling
- specific recommendations on the big and small nutrients

Over the last few decades, the American Diabetes Association (ADA) has revised its nutrition principles and recommendations for healthy eating numerous times. ADA's goal is to have these recommendations reflect the most current diabetes and nutrition research, as well as consensus among diabetes nutrition experts. Find and read the most current ADA nutrition recommendations at www.diabetes.org.

As you review these recommendations, you will see how similar they are to the Dietary Guidelines discussed in chapter 3. You'll also note that the focus of diabetes care is much broader than just attending to blood glucose control. Today, diabetes care includes managing blood glucose, blood lipid, and blood pressure levels. Keeping these three factors in the target ranges (see ABC goals on page 5) will keep you healthy for years to come.

Healthy Eating with Diabetes

Here are four key principles to remember about healthy eating with diabetes:

1. **There's no such thing as a "diabetic diet."** These so-called diabetic diets shouldn't be used. The healthy eating guidelines for everyone apply to people with diabetes as well. People with diabetes do not need to buy or eat any special foods.

2. **Change your behaviors slowly but surely.** Healthy eating and staying active are well-known and effective ways to stay healthy. They are essential if you are at high risk of type 2 diabetes, or have pre-diabetes or type 2 diabetes because you are more likely to have or be at high risk for heart and blood vessel diseases. When you learn that you have type 2 diabetes, your eating habits and food choices may need changing.

● QUICK TIP

Try not to think of your eating plan as a "diet." Think of it as a way to slowly change your family's eating habits for the better.

3. **Individualization is important.** Find a registered dietitian (RD) who specializes in diabetes medical nutrition therapy (MNT). Medical nutrition therapy is the formal name for nutrition counseling. It is the term some health plans, including Medicare, use to describe coverage of nutrition counseling. Your RD should work with you to develop a personalized healthy eating plan and goals for behavior change. This health care provider should consider all of your health, diabetes, and nutrition goals, as well as your food preferences: including what foods you like to eat; what time you like to eat; your cultural and religious food habits and customs; whether you like or need snacks at certain times; your daily and weekend schedule; and, most important, what you are willing, able, and ready to change. For instance, the eating plan and goals for a vegetarian who works the evening shift would be very different from those of someone who lives alone and eats most meals in restaurants.

4. **Be flexible and realistic with yourself.** In today's fast-paced world, life doesn't always go according to plan, and the healthiest foods are not always at your disposal. Your eating plan and behavior change goals need to be flexible enough to fit your lifestyle. They need to help you be able to delay a meal or snack, eat at a restaurant, or opt for convenience foods. Your eating plan needs to fit the days when your activity level is way up—perhaps for a weekend hike or day of skiing—and the days when you feel ill and have no appetite.

Recommendations for Big and Small Nutrients

Most people at high risk for or with type 2 diabetes need to shed some weight. To lose those 10 to 20 pounds, you need to know the right number of calories for you to eat, along with the proper foods that will provide the right mix of carbohydrate, protein, and fat. Research shows there is no single combination of nutrients that's best for diabetes care and/or weight control.

The goals below give a calorie range to shoot for when it comes to each of the big nutrients.

Carbohydrate

Carbohydrate is the main nutrient that raises blood glucose levels. Both the amount and the type of carbohydrate you eat will affect your blood glucose, but the amount has a greater effect on your blood glucose. Once you learn the impact of carbohydrate on blood glucose, it's rational to think that a low carbohydrate intake may be an answer to blood glucose control. Research doesn't support this notion. Many studies have shown that a lower carbohydrate intake can help lower blood glucose initially; however, over time, it doesn't improve weight loss, blood glucose control, and most other health parameters of interest. Lower carbohydrate diets (less than 45% of calories from carbohydrate) also don't allot sufficient grams of carbohydrate to get the nutrients, fiber, vitamins, and minerals you need.

The ADA suggests that people with diabetes consult the general nutrition guidelines, which recommend that you get somewhere between 45 and 65% of your daily calories from carbohydrate. For example, suppose you eat about 1,400 calories a day and you decide to get half of those calories from carbohydrates. Because each gram of carbohydrate contains 4 calories, you would need to eat about 175 grams of carbohydrate to consume half of your total calories from carbohydrate. (In other words, half of 1,400 calories is 700, and 700 calories divided by 4 calories per gram is 175 grams.)

● **QUICK TIP**

It's important to eat similar amounts of carbohydrate at each meal and to keep snacks, if you need them, consistent.

If you are not able to keep your blood glucose levels on target by eating a healthy and balanced amount of carbohydrate throughout the day, you may need one or more blood glucose–lowering medications. Decreasing the amount of carbohydrate you eat to unhealthy levels will not bring your blood glucose down sufficiently. If you are not reaching your blood glucose goals, talk with your health care provider about the steps you should take to hit your blood glucose targets.

Sugars and Sweets

Sugars and sweets are no longer off-limits for people with diabetes. You can choose to fit sugars and sweets into your eating plan in small quantities; however, don't forget that they are concentrated sources of carbohydrate and calories and can elevate your blood glucose levels. Plus, sweets such as cheesecake and regular ice cream may be high in total fats, especially the unhealthy saturated fats. Finally, because sweets usually offer little in the way of nutrition, everyone who wants to eat healthier should limit the amount of sugars and sweets they eat. Consider your weight, blood glucose and blood fat levels, and diabetes goals when fitting sweets into your eating plan.

Dietary Fiber

In general, you should try to increase the amount of fiber you eat to 14 grams of fiber for every 1,000 calories you eat. The recommended daily fiber intake levels can help you figure out specifically how much fiber you should include in your diet.

These goals are roughly double the amount of fiber that most Americans eat (11–17 grams/day). Good sources of fiber are whole grains, beans and peas, fruits, and vegetables. You can get about 5 grams

Recommended Daily Fiber Intake	
Gender and Age	Amount (grams/day)
Men, age 50 and younger	38
Men, age 50 and older	30
Women, age 50 and younger	25
Women, age 50 and older	21

of dietary fiber from a serving of a whole-grain cereal, a third of a cantaloupe, or 1/2 cup of cooked lentils. Learn more about how to increase your fiber intake in section 2.

Glycemic Index and Glycemic Load

The use of the glycemic index (GI) and glycemic load (GL) in diabetes meal planning has been an area of debate for several decades. The ADA suggests that GI and GL may be valuable concepts for people with diabetes if these measures are used in addition to and after careful monitoring of total carbohydrate intake; however, using GI or GL to choose foods may or may not help you make healthier food choices. For example, you might decide to eat lentils or barley instead of white rice because lentils and barley have a lower glycemic index. Conversely, choosing a high-fat food like ice cream because it had a low GI instead of a serving of fruit with a higher GI, a banana or fresh pineapple, doesn't make sense. Think of GI and GL as another factor, rather than the main factor, to consider when you choose which foods to eat.

The GI measures the increase in blood glucose levels during the two hours after eating a particular kind of food. Some foods that contain carbohydrate create a quick and more dramatic rise in blood glucose, while others cause a slower and less dramatic rise. Glucose is the standard for the glycemic index and is assigned an arbitrary number of 100. Other foods are assigned GI numbers relative to the glucose standard of 100—either higher or lower. Today, there are several different glycemic indexes in use.

Keep in mind that GI numbers are available only for several hundred commonly eaten, non-mixed foods. In other words, foods like carrots, watermelon, and potatoes have GI numbers, but casseroles and vegetable soup do not. It's also important to note that the type of carbohydrate (e.g., starch or sugar) does not consistently predict the GI. For example, some fruits have a low GI and others have a higher GI. The GI doesn't consider typical food portions; however, GL does. The GL takes the glycemic index of a food and then factors in its common serving sizes to give a more practical indicator of the effect that food will have on blood glucose.

Raising Your Blood Glucose

Other factors that contribute to how foods raise your blood glucose are

- your blood glucose at the time you eat
- how much blood glucose–lowering medicine you take, when you take it, and when you eat
- your level of insulin resistance in general and at the time you eat the food(s)
- individual responses to foods and different responses on different days
- the amount of fiber and whole grains in a meal (these can slow the rise of blood glucose)
- how ripe a fruit or vegetable is when you eat it (the riper the food, the more quickly it can raise blood glucose)
- the form of the food (for example, fettuccine can affect blood glucose differently than macaroni)
- the variety of the food (for example, long-grain or short-grain rice, Yukon gold or red potatoes, and when and where a product was grown)
- whether you eat the food raw or cooked (the more a food is cooked, the more likely it is to raise blood glucose quickly)
- the other foods you eat along with the carbohydrate (a meal that is mainly carbohydrate with a small amount of fat will raise your blood glucose more quickly than a meal with more fat)

Many of the foods that have a low GI are healthy foods. Consider eating more whole-grain breads and cereals, legumes (beans), and fruits and vegetables. Include these foods in your eating plan, but don't completely omit foods with a higher GI if they are healthy foods and you enjoy them.

You may find it helpful to create your own personal GI by recording the results of your after-meal blood glucose checks. Make notes about your experiences with certain foods and meals, and note what changes you might make when you eat that food or meal again, such as eating a smaller portion, avoiding them, or adjusting medicine (if you can).

Consider using the concepts of GI and GL in conjunction with other healthy eating strategies and priorities. First, look at your total carbohydrate count at meals, limit your intake of sweets and sugars, increase the amount of whole grains, fruits, and vegetables you eat, and then factor in the GI or GL of a food.

Protein

The ADA suggests that eating 15–20% of your calories as protein is fine as long as you don't have diabetes-related kidney disease. This is not a lot of protein, as you can see in the model meals on pages 53–58. Eating 15–20% of your calories as protein certainly doesn't allow for an 8-ounce piece of steak, fish, or chicken each night at dinner. Eating smaller (about 2–4 ounces), as well as leaner, portions of animal protein will also help reduce your intake of saturated and trans fat and will help you to reach your blood lipid targets. Read the information on fat, below, to learn more.

Protein can influence blood glucose, but to a much lesser degree than carbohydrate does. In people with type 2 who still make some insulin on their own, protein intake can cause an increase in the release of insulin from the pancreas; however, this doesn't raise blood glucose. Because people with type 1 diabetes no longer make insulin, moderate amounts of protein have little effect on blood glucose. Keep in mind that a high-protein meal, which is often also high in fat, can cause a delayed rise in blood glucose.

> ● **QUICK TIP**
>
> Most Americans eat more protein than their bodies need to be healthy— about 15–20% of your total calories. Portions need to be closer to 2–4 ounces cooked to achieve this goal.

Fat

As a person with diabetes or pre-diabetes, you may have abnormal blood lipid levels (unhealthy LDL, low HDL, and/or high triglycerides) and high blood pressure. Because these conditions put you at risk for heart and blood vessel problems, the most important advice for you is to limit the amount of saturated fat you eat to less than 7% of calories and to keep trans fat as low as possible. In years past, there was more emphasis on eating less total fat. Today, experts believe that anywhere from about 20–40% of your calories can come from fat. The key is to minimize the unhealthy fats and oils and to get the remainder of your calories from fat from the healthier monounsaturated and polyunsaturated fats. With our food choices today this is easier said than done. Try to keep your trans fat intake as close to zero as possible.

Fat affects blood glucose by slowing down the rise of blood glucose after you eat. In other words, a high-fat meal may cause a slower rise in blood glucose than a high-carbohydrate meal. This doesn't mean you should eat a lot of fat, especially saturated fat, as a way to manage your blood glucose. Keep your total fat intake moderate and choose the healthiest fats. You'll learn how to reach these goals in the pages ahead.

Sodium

Research showing the benefits of a lower sodium count on blood pressure is mounting. Control of blood pressure is an important topic because nearly three-quarters of people with diabetes have high blood pressure. A lower sodium intake can impact blood pressure even more in people with diabetes or high blood pressure, along with African Americans and adults who are middle-aged and older. Keep in mind that we now eat around 4,000–6,000 milligrams of sodium a day. More than half of this is from processed foods. Research shows you can further lower your blood pressure by eating sufficient fruits, vegetables, whole grains, and low-fat dairy foods that provide much needed potassium (among other essential nutrients). Learn more about how to reduce your sodium intake and raise your potassium count in chapter 8.

● **QUICK TIP**

Research shows that getting your sodium intake down to below 2,500 milligrams per day can help lower and control blood pressure.

Alcohol

The recommendation for alcohol is consistent with general dietary guidelines. Women should have no more than 1 drink a day, and men should have no more than 2 drinks a day. Research shows there are some benefits of various types of alcohol on the heart.

Vitamins and Minerals

If you eat at least 1,200 calories a day from a wide variety of healthy foods and your blood glucose levels are within the target ranges at this point, the ADA does not believe you need to take vitamin, mineral, or dietary supplements. People with diabetes have not been shown to have any greater need for various vitamins and minerals than anyone else.

You may be at risk for or have difficulty getting sufficient amounts of some critical vitamins and minerals. Studies show that many people are deficient in vitamins A, C, D, and E along with essential minerals like choline, folic acid, magnesium, and potassium. Your first step to ensure that you do get enough of these important nutrients is to eat a wide variety of foods. Choose nutrient-rich as well as minimally processed foods. Next, talk to your health care provider about a multivitamin and mineral supplement that offers you optimal amounts of missing vitamins and minerals as extra "insurance." This is especially true if your daily calorie intake is at or below 1,200, or you know you don't get enough of certain vitamins or minerals. (See chapter 7 for more information on vitamins, minerals, and supplements.)

Vegetarianism and Diabetes

Vegetarianism has exploded across the country in the last several years. There are more restaurants that cater to the vegetarian and vegan lifestyle. If you're a vegetarian or thinking about becoming a vegetarian and you're worried that it won't mesh with your diabetes healthy eating lifestyle, think again. There is no reason a person with diabetes can't adopt a vegetarian lifestyle.

● Q U I C K   T I P

The nutrients vegetarians need to be concerned about are those provided by meats, poultry, and seafood as well as dairy products and eggs (if these are omitted). Consider your intake of calcium, iron, zinc, vitamin B-12, vitamin D, riboflavin, and omega-3 fats. Discuss the use of vitamin and mineral supplementation with your care providers.

Being a vegetarian represents a broad range of eating styles. Some vegetarians do not eat any meat products but will still consume milk and eggs, while vegans restrict all animal products from their diet. Others do not eat red meat, but will occasionally eat seafood or poultry. The Vegetarian Resource Group (www.vrg.org) defines four categories of vegetarianism.

Research shows that vegetarians tend to receive a multitude of health benefits because of their higher consumption of foods from healthier food groups, along with fiber and other nutrients; however, just because someone is a vegetarian doesn't mean they automatically eat more healthfully. Vegetarians need to work just as hard (if not harder) to choose healthy foods and eat them in healthful ways. It will be important to choose and prepare your foods with limited fats and salt (as suggested for everyone) and to monitor your ABCs to make sure you are hitting your targets. If your blood glucose is difficult to control, you may be ready for blood glucose–lowering medication.

Health Benefits of Vegetarianism

Proven health benefits for those people who practice a vegetarian lifestyle are:

- Lower LDL cholesterol
- Lower blood pressure
- Lower rates of type 2 diabetes (over non-vegetarians)
- Lower body weight

Chapter 5

Secrets of Successful Weight Loss and Control

What You'll Learn:

- realistic weight loss goals
- how weight loss can improve your ABCs
- an optimal eating plan for weight control
- secrets of successful long-term weight control
- whether weight loss medications or gastric surgery can be effective

During the last decade, much has been learned about the impact of weight loss on health and preventing or managing type 2 diabetes. Research studies have also revealed how people can succeed at losing weight and keeping that weight off over time. Bottom line: It takes a lot more doing than knowing when it comes to short- and long-term weight control.

Be Realistic about Weight Loss

For most people, it's neither realistic nor necessary to get back down to the weight you were when you were a teen or young adult. This is especially true if you've become overweight or obese. Losing weight and keeping it off is tough for everyone for several reasons. People who lose weight seem to require fewer calories to maintain their lighter weight. There are also adaptations of hormones related to hunger and appetite control. Lastly, it appears that the presence of insulin resistance (a problem most people with pre-diabetes and type 2 have) makes weight loss and control even tougher.

● QUICK TIP

Keep in mind any weight you lose is a move in the right direction. It's worth noting that on average, an adult puts on two pounds a year, so, just preventing further weight gain is an accomplishment!

Research shows that you'll be more successful if you lose a small amount of weight (10 to 20 pounds) and work hard to maintain this healthier weight. Numerous studies show that your weight loss will be greatest at six months. If you want to lose a few more pounds, try it several months later; however, remember that maintaining the initial weight loss is what's most important for your long-term diabetes control.

Weight Loss and Blood Glucose Control

For many years, it was believed that many people with diabetes could control their blood glucose with a healthy eating plan, weight loss, and by increasing physical activity. This notion no longer stands up to research for many people. Some people can control their blood glucose for a time if their type 2 diabetes is detected early (or if pre-diabetes is diagnosed), and they are diligent about implementing a healthy eating plan, etc.

Weight loss accomplished by healthy eating and physical activity can decrease insulin resistance, improve insulin sensitivity, and result in lower blood glucose, lower blood pressure, and improved blood lipids for a time.

You and your provider will be able to determine if healthier lifestyle habits and weight loss are effectively controlling your blood glucose anywhere from six weeks to three months after you start to change your lifestyle habits. For most people with type 2 diabetes, lifestyle changes and weight loss, though beneficial for a variety of reasons, will not be substantial enough to control blood glucose over time. By the time you are diagnosed or decide to take action, you may have had type 2 for years and your insulin-making capacity may have dwindled by 50 to 80%. Weight loss alone is unlikely to sufficiently improve blood glucose numbers. This doesn't mean that you've failed, it means that your type 2 diabetes is progressing.

ADA recommendations suggest that most people diagnosed with diabetes be started on a blood glucose–lowering medication like metformin at diagnosis. There is no doubt that healthy eating, being physically active, and keeping your weight down will help any medication work more efficiently to help you control your ABCs over time.

Optimal Eating Plan for Weight Control

Research over the past few years points to the conclusion that the best eating plan for weight loss is one that fits your food and cultural preferences and one that you can follow comfortably for years to come. Sufficient research on low carbohydrate diets suggests that people can't follow these plans any more effectively than high-carbohydrate (>50%), low-fat (<30%) plans. A large two-year study published in early 2009 showed that overweight people who were on a variety of diets gradually gravitated back to a carbohydrate range of 43–53%, within the range of current carbohydrate recommendations.

Secrets of Successful Weight Control

With the combination of research results and several studies of large groups of people who have lost weight and kept it off, the secrets of weight control success are emerging. Keeping weight off takes discipline and persistence and implementation of these successful strategies.

- Slowly change your food and activity habits.
- Put together an eating plan that considers your food preferences.
- Focus on eating less fat. Eat no more than 25–30% of your calories as fat.
- Get and stay physically active (the most common form of activity is walking) at least 30 minutes a day. Have a realistic and achievable weight-loss goal in mind.
- Incorporate sufficient dietary fiber in your eating plan. This includes fruits, vegetables, and whole grains.
- Eat breakfast every day. It gets you off to a healthy start and revs your metabolism.
- Consider the use of meal replacements (bars, meals, soups, drinks) that are calorie- and portion-controlled foods.
- Weigh yourself at least once a week, if not more.
- Watch less than 10 hours of TV per week.
- Keep records of various aspects of your plan. Record keeping continues to prove valuable in maximizing success.
- Maintain frequent and ongoing contact with a health care provider, behavioral counselor, or other support system.

Learn more at the National Weight Control Registry, www.nwcr.ws.

What about Weight Loss Medications?

Today, there are only a couple of weight loss medications approved by the Food and Drug Administration (FDA)—sibutramine (Meridia) and orlistat (Xenical). Orlistat is now available over-the-counter in a low dose formula called Alli. Research studies do not generally show that any of these medications greatly improve weight loss or long-term control. They may help give some people an extra boost as part of a healthy lifestyle plan. Keep your eyes open for many other weight-loss medications, which are in the drug pipeline.

Obesity Treatment with Surgery

There's growing interest in the use of several bariatric surgical techniques to put pre-diabetes and type 2 diabetes into remission. These surgeries are referred to as bariatric, gastric or metabolic surgery; and have the potential to promote significant weight loss and control of blood glucose in obese people with pre-diabetes and type 2 diabetes. The surgeries most successful for pre-diabetes or type 2 diabetes reroute the intestines to avoid the duodenum (first section of the small intestine).

Any type of gastric surgery should be done within a program that offers a comprehensive approach to care. This means that pre- and post-surgical medical, psychological, and nutrition counseling are included. Some health plans and Medicare require that the surgery be done at a Center of Excellence. This status is achieved through the American Society for Metabolic and Bariatric Surgery and can be found at http://www.surgical review.org/locate.aspx.

Interestingly, the success of gastric surgery appears to be beyond simply helping people

> ● **QUICK TIP**
>
> The decision to have gastric surgery is a life-changing decision and shouldn't be entered into lightly. It will require significant changes in your eating habits and lifestyle.

lose more weight with relative speed. It appears that these surgeries have an important impact on correcting abnormalities of hormones involved with appetite, hunger, and blood glucose control.

The ADA suggests that people with type 2 diabetes whose body mass index (BMI) is at or greater than 35 can consider discussing bariatric surgery with their health care provider as a means to achieve weight loss and metabolic control. However, ADA strongly notes that people who have one of these surgeries will need lifelong support and medical monitoring.

Learn more

- www. win.niddk.nih.gov/publications/gastric.htm—Weight Control Information Network (NIH)
- www.asmbs.org—American Society for Metabolic and Bariatric Surgery
- www.acsbscn.org—American College of Surgeons Bariatric Surgery Center Network

Chapter

Personalize Your Healthy Eating Plan

What You'll Learn:

- the best calorie range for you
- the main food groups
- the number of servings to eat each day from each main food group based on your calorie needs
- how to divide your calories and food servings into meals and snacks
- how to plan meals and snacks within the calories you need each day, with several samples

In previous chapters, you've learned the general guidelines for healthy eating, as well as the specifics on healthy eating with diabetes. You've also seen that these messages about healthy eating are very similar and that their intention is to get and keep you healthy. This chapter helps you learn how to create a healthy eating plan that works for your lifestyle.

The Right Calories for You

You might wonder how many calories you need each day. The answer depends on many factors:

- your age and sex
- how active you are
- whether you want to lose or gain weight or stay at the same weight
- whether you have lost and gained weight many times or this is your first effort, and more.

The chart on page 48 can help you figure out how many calories and servings of various types of foods you need each day. Servings of food, for the purposes of this book, are defined in the tables provided at the end of each food group chapter in section 2. These servings are in sync with those in *Choose Your Foods: Exchange Lists for Diabetes* compiled by the American Dietetic Association and the American Diabetes Association. Note that these food servings may be different from those used on food packages or in other serving definitions.

These meal plans contain about 50% of calories from carbohydrate, 20% from protein, and 30% from fat. These percentages fall into the ranges suggested for healthy eating. They also reflect the way many people split their calories.

Here are some other factors to keep in mind when using the chart on page 48 to figure your calorie needs:

- **Use calorie ranges as a general guide only.** To learn how many calories and other nutrients you need to achieve your

diabetes and nutrition goals, work with a dietitian who specializes in diabetes.

- **Your activity level affects the amount of calories you need.** A
sedentary lifestyle is defined as one that includes only the light
physical activity you do to complete the daily tasks of life, such
as getting to work, doing laundry, fixing meals, and so on. An
active lifestyle includes physical activity equal to walking more
than 3 miles a day at 3 to 4 miles per hour, in addition to the
activities of daily living.

- **Some older women who are small in stature and sedentary
may need to eat no more than 1,200 calories to lose weight.**
At 1,200 calories, however, you may need a vitamin and mineral supplement to meet your nutrition needs.

- **The servings and calculations in the milk group are based on
fat-free milk.** Children between 9 and 18 years of age need
1,300 mg of calcium per day. They should get at least 3 servings
of milk per day. Adults ages 19 to 50 need 1,000 mg of calcium
per day. You can meet this goal with 2 servings of milk a day
plus another serving of a high-calcium food. Women over age
50 need 1,200 mg of calcium per day. To make up for the carbohydrate in 2 cups of milk, add 24 grams from starches, nonstarchy vegetables, or fruit.

- **The calories and nutrient information for meats are based
on average figures for lean meat (7 grams of protein and 3
grams of fat per ounce).** Adjust the grams or servings of fat
based on the type of meats you tend to eat. Choose lean sources
of meat and meat substitutes as often as possible (see chapter 13 for more information). Consult with your health care
providers if you have questions about your daily calorie needs.

Be Realistic! Aim for a Calorie Range

The actual calories you eat are not exact and greatly depend on the
fat content of the foods you choose. One day, you might be on the
low side because you chose grilled chicken or fish and ate vegetables

Figure Your Calorie Range and Food Servings

Find Your Calorie Range

Which category fits you?	Women who... • want to lose weight • are small in size and/or are sedentary	Women who... • are older and smaller • are larger and want to lose weight • and/or are sedentary	Women who... • are moderate to large size Men who... • are older • are small to moderate size and want to lose weight	Children Teen girls Women who... • are larger size and active Men who... • are small to moderate size and are at desired body weight	Teen boys Men who... • are active and moderate to large size
Daily calorie range	1,200–1,400	1,400–1,600	1,600–1,900	1,900–2,300	2,300–2,800

Figure Your Servings from Each Food Group

Starches	6	7	8	11	13
Vegetables (nonstarchy)	3	4	4	5	5
Fruits	3	3	3	4	5
Milk and yogurt	2	2	2	2	2
Meat and meat substitutes	4 oz	5 oz	6 oz	7 oz	8 oz
Fats	6	6	8	9	12

with little to no added fats. The next day the opposite may be true because you're dining out and choosing a higher-fat meat or adding dessert to your meal. Another big factor is how exact you are about your portions. Research shows that people can be off in their calorie counts by 500 calories at the end of a day simply by eating a little more than they realized, or guessing portions rather than weighing and measuring them precisely.

Your main goal, over the course of a week or month, is to average out your target calorie level. If you eat a few higher-fat choices one day, choose lower-fat choices the next. Over the long-term, change your eating habits and make healthier food choices to improve your diabetes management. Remember to focus your behavior changes on healthy eating strategies.

The Food Groups

This book groups foods into six main groups. Foods are divided into these groups based on the nutrients they provide and their effect on blood glucose levels. Grouping foods this way makes it easier for you to put together and eat healthy meals. You'll learn much more about each food group in the chapters in section 2.

- **Starch:** This group includes all foods made from grains, such as bread, hot and dry cereal, rice, pasta, and crackers. The group also contains starchy vegetables like potatoes, corn, peas, and legumes (beans). You should aim to eat at least three servings of foods made from whole grain each day. It is also important to pack plenty of dietary fiber into the starches you choose.
- **Vegetables:** This group includes all fresh, frozen, and canned vegetables and vegetable juices. Note that the starchy vegetables are in the starch food group. Consider the vegetables in this group nonstarchy.
- **Fruits:** This group includes all fresh, frozen, canned, and dried fruits and fruit juices.

- **Milk and yogurt:** These foods are your best sources of calcium. Fat-free or low-fat milk and yogurt are the healthiest choices. Foods made from milk that have little or no calcium, such as cream cheese, cream, and butter, are generally found in the fat group. You'll find cheese, another good source of calcium, in the meat and meat substitute group.
- **Meat and meat substitutes:** This group includes meats, poultry, seafood, eggs, cheese, and peanut butter. These foods provide you with much of the protein you eat. Choose lean sources of protein and prepare them in low-fat ways.
- **Fats:** These are the fats and oils you use when you prepare or eat foods. The foods in this group include the oil that you sauté vegetables in, the margarine you spread on toast, salad dressings, nuts, and bacon.

Not included in these six basic groups are sugars and sweets and alcohol and other beverages (with or without calories).

From Servings to Meals and Snacks

The next step is to figure out how to divide your allotted servings of food into balanced and tasty meals and snacks. Eating three meals a day is the foundation of a healthy eating plan that will help you keep your blood glucose on target. Note the meal skipped most regularly, breakfast, is the one found to be most important in weight control! It's best not to skip meals, especially if you take a blood glucose–lowering medicine that can cause low blood glucose.

Snacks

People with diabetes used to be told to eat every few hours to make sure their blood glucose didn't get too low. Times have changed dramatically! Some people take one or more diabetes medications that don't cause low blood glucose, and some use a combination of long- and rapid-acting insulins that tend to cause fewer problems with hypoglycemia.

With these therapies the messages about the *need* to snack have changed. Snacks are not a must. You may *want* to include snacks because they help you achieve your diabetes and healthy eating goals, or you might be thrilled to do away with the bothersome preparation and toting of snacks.

Putting Together Your Plan

To plan which foods to eat at your meals and snacks, ask yourself these questions about your daily life:

- What foods do you enjoy, and when do you want to eat them?
- What is your schedule for your blood glucose–lowering medications?
- How often and at what times do you have low blood glucose (hypoglycemia)?
- How much do you like to eat at different meals and snacks?
- Do you want or need snacks?
- What other nutrients do you need to consider? For example, do you have concerns about sodium and blood pressure or saturated and trans fat and blood lipids?
- How often do you eat meals away from home, and what types of foods do you eat when you eat out?
- Do you take vitamin and mineral supplements? Which ones and how much?
- What is your weight history?
- What is your usual activity level?
- What is your usual life schedule? If you work, what are your work hours? How do your weekdays vary from weekends? Are there other regular events in your schedule to consider?

If you wonder whether to keep snacks in your eating plan or not, remember that you should include them only if

- you want them
- you need them to prevent your blood glucose from going too low even after you and your health care provider have adjusted your blood glucose–lowering medications to prevent hypoglycemia
- you need to include snacks to eat enough calories or get enough of certain nutrients (pertinent for young children, women who are pregnant, or people who are underweight or recovering from a medical problem or procedure).

Learn by Example

The following one-day sample meals for three different calorie ranges can help you translate the calories and food servings in the chart on page 48 into an eating plan you can put into action. These sample meals include a wide variety of foods, so you can choose from foods you prepare at home, convenience foods, and restaurant foods. The nutrients in each menu are provided in the Nutrition Facts format to make them easy to review.

The sample meal plan for 1,400–1,600 calories is used again in most of the chapters in section 2 to show you how to plan meals with the number of servings of food you need each day. Depending on the day, you will have slightly more or less calories and more or less of some nutrients. This depends entirely on your food choices, but as long as you consistently eat a wide variety of healthy foods and sufficient calories, you should get the right amounts of the nutrients you need over the course of a week.

Sample Meal Plan: 1,200–1,400 Calories

Daily Servings from Food Groups

6 starches	3 vegetables	3 fruits
2 milk & yogurt	4 oz meat	6 fats

BREAKFAST

1 cup oatmeal (cooked) with	2 starches
2 tsp ground flax seed and	free food
1 Tbsp raisins	1/2 fruit
1/2 cup fat-free milk	1/2 milk
1/2 cup plain nonfat yogurt with	1/2 milk
1/2 small banana, sliced	1/2 fruit

LUNCH

1/2 whole-wheat pita pocket (6 inch)	1 starch
2 oz salmon (canned) made with:	2 oz meat
2 tsp mayonnaise	2 fat
1/2 cup sliced cucumbers	1/2 vegetable
1/3 cup alfalfa sprouts	1/2 vegetable
1/4 avocado, sliced	1 fat
1 oz baked tortilla chips	1 starch
1 nectarine (5 oz)	1 fruit

DINNER

Chef salad	2 vegetables
1 1/2 cups romaine lettuce	
2 Tbsp chopped mushrooms	
1/3 cup canned beets	
1/3 cup fresh tomatoes	
1/2 cup sliced peaches, canned	1 fruit
2 oz roasted chicken	2 oz meat
2 tsp canola oil	2 fat
Vinegar	free food
Dinner roll, whole wheat with	1 starch
1 1/2 tsp tub margarine (no trans fat)	1 fat

(continues)

Sample Meal Plan: 1,200–1,400 Calories *(continued)*

EVENING SNACK

1 cup sugar-free hot cocoa from mix   1 milk
3 gingersnaps   1 starch

Nutrition Facts

Calories 1,395	Calories from Fat 405
	% of calories
Total Fat 45 g	**29%**
Saturated Fat 9 g	**6%**
Monounsaturated Fat 19 g	
Cholesterol 92 mg	
Sodium 1,487 mg	
Total Carbohydrate 198 g	**53%**
Dietary Fiber 27 g	
Protein 70 g	**18%**
Vitamin A 141% • Vitamin C 88%	
Calcium 98% • Iron 106%	

Sample Meal Plan: 1,400–1,600 Calories

Daily Servings from Food Groups

7 starches	4 vegetables	3 fruits
2 milk & yogurt	5 oz meat	6 fats

BREAKFAST

1/2 whole grain bagel (2 oz) with	2 starches
1 1/2 Tbsp light cream cheese	1 fat
3/4 cup blueberries with	1 fruit
1/3 cup plain fat-free yogurt	1/2 milk

LUNCH

Tuna salad made with:	
2 oz tuna (1/2 cup), water-packed	2 oz meat
1 Tbsp light mayonnaise	1 fat
2 Tbsp diced celery	1 vegetable
1 Tbsp diced onions	
Tomato slices	1 free food
2 slices whole-wheat bread	2 starches
1 cup raw or blanched broccoli	1 vegetable
1 cup fat-free milk	1 milk
1/2 large apple	1 fruit

DINNER

3 oz grilled salmon with	3 oz meat
lemon and herbs	free food
Stir-fried vegetables with:	
1/4 cup onions, cooked	2 vegetables
1/2 cup snow peas, cooked	
1/2 cup red peppers, cooked	
2 tsp canola oil	2 fats
1 cup brown rice	3 starches

(continues)

Sample Meal Plan: 1,400–1,600 Calories *(continued)*

EVENING SNACK

Mix together:

1/2 cup crushed canned pineapple (packed in own juice)	1 fruit
1/3 cup plain fat-free yogurt	1/2 milk
1/8 cup chopped pecans	2 fats

Nutrition Facts

Calories 1,550   **Calories from Fat** 459

% of calories

Total Fat 51 g — 28%

Saturated Fat 11 g — 7%

Monounsaturated Fat 21 g

Cholesterol 113 mg

Sodium 1,427 mg

Total Carbohydrate 207 g — 51%

Dietary Fiber 27 g

Protein 81 g — 21%

Vitamin A 152%   •   Vitamin C 338%

Calcium 87%   •   Iron 67%

Sample Meal Plan: 1,900–2,300 Calories

Daily Servings from Food Groups

11 starches	5 vegetables	4 fruits
2 milk & yogurt	7 oz meat	9 fats

BREAKFAST

1 fried egg with	1 oz meat
2 tsp light tub margarine	1 fat
2 slices whole-wheat toast with	2 starch
2 tsp low-sugar jelly	free food
1/2 pink grapefruit	1 fruit
1 cup fat-free milk	1 milk

LUNCH

Fast-food hamburger, plain (quarter pound) with ketchup and mustard	2 starches, 3 oz meat, 2 fat free food
1 order small French fries with ketchup (2 Tbsp)	2 starch, 2 fat free food
1 garden salad (large)	2 vegetable
2 tsp oil (2 fat) plus vinegar (free)	2 fat
2 4-oz tangerines (from home)	1 fruit

DINNER

1 cup turkey chili (homemade)	1 starch, 1 vegetable, 2 oz meat
1 medium baked potato (6 oz)	2 starch
1 oz grated low-fat cheese	1 oz meat, 1 fat
1/2 cup baby carrots	1 vegetable
1/2 cup sliced cucumbers	1 vegetable
2 Tbsp light ranch salad dressing for dip	1 fat
1 sliced kiwi (3 1/2 oz, large)	1 fruit

(continues)

Sample Meal Plan: 1,900–2,300 Calories *(continued)*

EVENING SNACK

3/4 cup bran flakes	1 starch
1/4 cup low-fat granola (no raisins)	1 starch
1 cup fat-free milk	1 milk
8 dried apricot halves	1 fruit

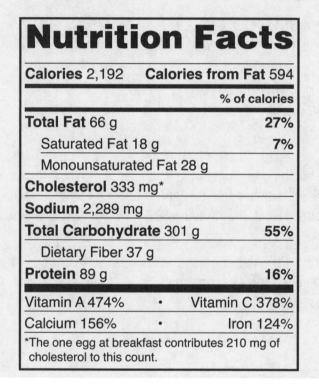

Nutrition Facts

Calories 2,192   **Calories from Fat** 594

% of calories

Total Fat 66 g	**27%**
Saturated Fat 18 g	**7%**
Monounsaturated Fat 28 g	
Cholesterol 333 mg*	
Sodium 2,289 mg	
Total Carbohydrate 301 g	**55%**
Dietary Fiber 37 g	
Protein 89 g	**16%**

Vitamin A 474%	•	Vitamin C 378%
Calcium 156%	•	Iron 124%

*The one egg at breakfast contributes 210 mg of cholesterol to this count.

Chapter 7

Vitamins, Minerals, and Dietary Supplements

What You'll Learn:

- the definitions for vitamins, minerals, and dietary supplements
- ADA recommendations on vitamins, minerals, and dietary supplements
- how to take a "foods first" approach to eat enough vitamins and minerals
- the intake recommendations (daily value) for vitamins and minerals
- top 10 food sources of key vitamins and minerals
- facts about dietary supplements of interest to people with diabetes
- factors to consider before you buy and try dietary supplements

Vitamins, Minerals, and Dietary Supplements Defined

Vitamins are essential substances contained in foods that help your body use the food you eat for proper functioning. Each vitamin performs unique tasks. Vitamins often partner with enzymes in your body to carry out specific tasks.

Minerals, like vitamins, are essential substances found in foods that help your body use the food you eat to make your body work properly. Each mineral serves a particular role. For example, calcium strengthens your bones, and potassium helps regulate the circulatory system and helps control blood pressure. Minerals often partner with enzymes in your body to accomplish certain tasks.

Dietary supplements include vitamins, minerals, herbs, botanicals, and other substances that perform, or claim to perform, actions in your body to achieve good health and/or prevent or control health problems. They are not food or drugs, but they contain one or more ingredients that are usually found in foods. They are intended to be used in addition to food, not as a replacement for a healthy eating plan. In the United States, the FDA regulates dietary supplements, but doesn't regulate the approval or marketing of supplements in the same manner as prescribed medicines. The FDA does not approve dietary supplements before they are allowed on the market, but it can take dietary supplements off the market if problems occur. The FDA now requires all supplement containers to be labeled "dietary supplement" and to have a Supplement Facts label that is similar in look, but not content, to the Nutrition Facts label on foods and beverages.

ADA Recommendations

If you eat a wide variety of nutrient-packed healthy foods, eat at least 1,200 calories a day, and generally keep your blood glucose within target goals, the ADA does not believe that you need to take vitamins, minerals, and/or dietary supplements to achieve optimal nutrient intake.

Many American adults and children don't get adequate amounts of several key nutrients for two main reasons: 1) inadequate intake of the foods packed with vitamins and minerals: fruits, vegetables, whole grains, low-fat dairy foods, and 2) inadequate availability of some nutrients in the common food supply.

If you think you may not be getting adequate supplies of vitamins and minerals, your first step

is to eat a wider variety of foods and to choose more nutrient-packed foods. If you still feel you have some "nutrition gaps," you may want to take a multivitamin and mineral supplement that offers a good supply of the vitamins and minerals you need; however, it is difficult to get sufficient amounts of some vitamins and minerals from a combination of foods and multivitamin supplements. For these nutrients, such as calcium and Vitamin D, you may need to take an individual supplement. (See the section on daily values, on page 63, for more information.)

Vitamin and Supplement Needs

The ADA does note that a person with diabetes may need a specific vitamin or mineral supplement if you

- are a strict vegetarian (meaning you eliminate a number of food groups)
- are following a weight-reducing meal plan of 1,200 calories or less per day
- are pregnant or breastfeeding
- are elderly
- have certain additional short- or long-term illnesses

If any of these factors apply to you, consider your current food intake and whether you are meeting your blood glucose goals.

The Missing Vitamins and Minerals

Nutrition intake surveys conducted by the U.S. government on a regular basis point out that while people are eating more calories per day than ever, about 2,150, we're falling short on certain key vitamins and minerals. A big reason for the shortfall: adults are not eating enough whole grains, fruits, and vegetables and are eating too much added sugars and fats. Adults are not consuming enough of vitamins A, C, D, E, and the minerals: calcium, choline, folate, potassium, and magnesium. Except for vitamins A (as carotenoids) and C, children are lacking in this same list. While it's not a vitamin or a mineral, one nutrient that's lacking in most people's diet is dietary fiber.

To have the best chance of getting the vitamins, minerals, and dietary fiber you need, eat a wide variety of nutrient-dense (packed with vitamins and minerals) foods, such as fruits, vegetables, whole grains, and low-fat dairy foods, lean meats, nuts, seeds, beans, and healthy liquid oils. The guidelines also recommend lightening up on foods that are low in nutrients and are contributing excessive calories. These are drinks with added sugars, sweets, candy, fried foods, high-fat meats, and whole-milk dairy foods.

Take a Foods First Approach

Plan your meals and snacks to eat a wide variety of nutrient-dense foods and get the vast majority of your vitamins and minerals from the foods you eat. Experts in nutrition believe that foods contain vitamins and minerals as well as many naturally occurring substances (some not yet even known) that may protect against chronic health problems.

If you are keeping your calorie level low (1,500 calories and below) to meet your diabetes and nutrition goals, you'll have to

> ● **QUICK TIP**
>
> Keep nutrition-packed fruits, such as berries, bananas, oranges, apples, grapefruit, and mangos in your refrigerator and rotate your fruit choices.

work even harder to eat all the nutrients you need. If you need to eat less than 1,500 calories a day, or you cannot eat a particular category of food, ask your health care provider whether you should take a multivitamin and mineral supplement or a supplement that contains the nutrients you are lacking. For example, many people need to take a supplement to get enough calcium and vitamin D. Luckily, these nutrients are often paired in one supplement.

Vitamin and Mineral Needs: Who Sets the Targets?

Vitamin and mineral deficiencies, which can result in diseases, were much more common several hundred years ago. Today, people don't often get scurvy from having insufficient vitamin C, beriberi from a deficiency of thiamin, or rickets from not getting enough vitamin D. For the past few decades, government agencies and government-appointed experts have worked to establish which vitamins and minerals are necessary for health and how much of these vitamins and minerals people need at various ages and stages of life.

The recommendations for many vitamins and minerals are based on the Dietary Reference Intakes (DRIs), which are developed through the Institute of Medicine at the National Academy of Sciences. Over time, the DRIs are reviewed and revised based on the evolving nutrition science.

Daily Values on the Nutrition Facts Label

The Nutrition Facts label uses the single term Daily Value (DV) to provide nutrient levels, which will cover the needs of most people. The Daily Values provide food manufacturers with guidelines to follow for food labeling and nutrition claims. Keep in mind that Daily Values are based on a calorie intake of 2,000 calories a day.

The table on page 65 lists current Daily Values and the amount of the vitamin or mineral that a food must have per serving to use an "excellent source of" or "good source of" nutrition claim.

- The terms "excellent source of," "rich in," and "high" mean that a serving (noted on the food label) of the food provides 20% or more of the Daily Value.
- The terms "good source of," "contains," and "provides" mean that a serving of the food must provide 10–19% of the Daily Value.

Learn more about food labeling and use of the Nutrition Facts label in chapter 22.

Getting Enough Vitamins and Minerals

While the vitamin and mineral needs of people with diabetes are no different from those of other Americans, research shows that many adults don't get enough of the essential vitamins and minerals. These tips can help you:

- Eat more fruits and vegetables and eat a wide variety of them. Go for the high-color ones because they often provide more vitamins and minerals—orange, dark green, blue, and red.
- Eat more fruits and vegetables raw, unprocessed or minimally processed.
- Make many of your starch choices whole-wheat or whole grains—cereals and breads, brown rice, whole-wheat pasta, bulgur, and barley.
- Use legumes (beans, peas, and lentils) frequently. Make soups or bean salads or sprinkle beans or peas on tossed salad. These foods are packed with vitamins and minerals.
- Eat or drink 2 to 3 servings a day of low-fat milk, yogurt, or cheese. Many children and young adults don't get enough calcium and vitamin D. Dairy foods naturally contain calcium and are nearly always fortified with vitamin D.

Daily Values for Vitamins and Minerals with Levels for "Excellent Source" and "Good Source" Claims

Nutrient	Daily Value (based on 2,000 calories/day)	Excellent Source (20% or higher)	Good Source (10–19%)
Dietary Fiber	25 g	5 g	2.5–5 g
Sodium	2,400 mg	480 mg	240–456 mg
Potassium	3,500 mg	700 mg	350–665 mg
Vitamin A	5,000 IU	1,000 IU	500–950 IU
Vitamin C	60 mg	12 mg	6–11 mg
Calcium	1,000 mg	200 mg	100–190 mg
Iron	18 mg	3.6 mg	1.8–3.4 mg
Vitamin D	400 IU	80 IU	40–76 IU
Vitamin E	30 IU	6 IU	3–5.7 IU
Vitamin K	80 mcg	16 mcg	8–15.2 mcg
Thiamin	1.5 mg	0.3 mg	0.15–0.29 mg
Riboflavin	1.7 mg	0.34 mg	0.17–0.32 mg
Niacin	20 mg	4 mg	2–3.8 mg
Vitamin B6	2 mg	0.4 mg	0.2–0.38 mg
Folate	400 mcg	80 mcg	40–76 mcg
Vitamin B12	6.0 mcg	1.2 mcg	0.6–1.14 mcg
Biotin	300 mcg	60 mcg	30–57 mcg
Pantothenic acid	10 mg	2 mg	1–1.9 mg
Phosphorus	1,000 mg	200 mg	100–190 mg
Iodine	150 mcg	30 mcg	15–29 mcg
Magnesium	400 mg	80 mg	40–76 mg
Zinc	15 mg	3 mg	1.5–2.9 mg
Copper	2.0 mg	0.4 mg	0.2–0.38 mg
Selenium	70 mcg	14 mcg	7–13.3 mcg
Manganese	2.0 mg	0.4 mg	0.2–0.38 mg
Chromium	120 mcg	24 mcg	12–22.8 mcg
Molybdenum	75 mcg	15 mcg	7.5–14 mcg
Chloride	3,400 mg	680 mg	340–646 mg

Note: g = grams, mg = milligrams, IU = International Units, mcg = micrograms.

See the individual chapters in section 2 for more tips on how to eat your vitamins and minerals.

Top 10 for 10 Vitamins and Minerals

Each of the 10 tables on the following pages provides a list of the top 10 food sources (based on one serving of food) of the nutrients you are most likely to be lacking. At the top of each table, you'll find the daily value for each nutrient and the amount needed for a food to be considered an "excellent source" or a "good source" of the nutrient. Use these tables to see how the foods you eat stack up and to find new nutrition-packed foods to add to your eating plan. Nutrient data was obtained from the USDA nutrient database. This is a searchable database which is an excellent resource for nutrition information on about 8,000 foods at: www.ars.usda.gov/ba/bhnrc/ndl.

Vitamin D: Top Ten Food Sources Daily Value = 400 IU Excellent Source = 80 IU, Good Source = 40–76 IU			
Food	Serving	Food Group	Amount (IU)
Sardines, canned in oil	3 oz	Meat	429
Salmon, cooked	3 oz	Meat	300
Mackerel	3 oz	Meat	296
Tuna, canned	3 oz	Meat	200
Milk, fat free fortified	8 oz	Milk	100
Milk, 1%, fortified	8 oz	Milk	98
Orange juice, fortified	4 oz	Fruit	40
Cereal, dry flakes, fortified with 10% vitamin D	3/4 cup	Starch	40
Egg, whole, large	1	Meat	20
Margarine, fortified	1 tsp	Fat	20

Fiber: Top Ten Food Sources Daily Value = 25 g Excellent Source = 5 g Good Source = 2.5–5 g			
Food	Serving	Food Group	Amount (g)
Bran cereal (i.e., All-Bran, 100% Bran, Fiber One; some contain even extra fiber)	1/2 cup	Starch	10–18
Acorn or butternut squash, cooked	1 cup	Starch	6–8
Dried peas, beans, and lentils	1/2 cup	Starch	5–8
Bran flakes	3/4 cup	Starch	4–6
Raspberries	1 cup	Fruit	5
Blueberries	3/4 cup	Fruit	4
Brussels sprouts, cooked	1/2 cup	Vegetable	4
Corn, cooked	1/2 cup	Starch	4
Broccoli, spinach, or other greens	1/2 cup	Vegetable	3
Apricots, dried	8 halves	Fruit	3

Vitamin A: Top Ten Food Sources
Daily Value = 5,000 IU
Excellent Source = 1,000 IU   Good Source = 500–950 IU

Food	Serving	Food Group	Amount (IU)
Leafy greens, spinach, collards, or kale, cooked	1/2 cup	Vegetable	7,700–10,500
Liver, beef, or chicken, cooked	3 oz	Meat	5,200–8,900
Sweet potato	1/2 cup	Starch	3,682
Pumpkin, canned	3/4 cup	Starch	3,602
Red pepper, sliced	1 cup	Vegetable	2,881
Salmon, cooked	3 oz	Meat	2,826
Carrots, raw or cooked	1/2 cup	Vegetable	1,970
Cantaloupe	1/3	Fruit	1,565
Squash, winter	1 cup	Starch	1,435
Whole-grain cereal, cold	3/4 cup	Starch	855

Vitamin C: Top Ten Food Sources
Daily Value = 60 mg
Excellent Source = 12 mg   Good Source = 6–11 mg

Food	Serving	Food Group	Amount (mg)
Red pepper, sliced	1 cup	Vegetable	284
Strawberries	1 1/4 cups, sliced	Fruit	106
Kiwi	1 whole, 3.5 oz	Fruit	70
Orange	1	Fruit	70
Cantaloupe	1/3 melon, small	Fruit	67
Green pepper	1 cup	Vegetable	60
Grapefruit	1/2	Fruit	46
Papaya	1/2 whole	Fruit	43
Honeydew	1 cup	Fruit	42
Tomato or vegetable juice	1/2 cup	Vegetable	26

Vitamin E: Top Ten Food Sources
Daily Value = 30 IU*
Excellent Source = 6 IU   Good Source = 3–5.7 IU

Food	Serving	Food Group	Amount (IU)
Salad dressing, regular or reduced calorie	1 Tbsp	Fat	2.7–7.5
Peanut butter	2 Tbsp	Fat	6.4
Sweet potato	1/2 cup	Starch	7.6
Almonds	1 Tbsp	Fat	5.3
Whole-grain cereal, cold	3/4 cup	Starch	4.0–8.7
Sunflower seeds	1 Tbsp	Fat	4.7
Vegetable oils: sunflower, cottonseed, or canola	1 tsp	Fat	2.6–4.7
Spinach	1/2 cup	Vegetable	2.8
Whole-wheat dinner roll	1 roll	Starch	3.8
Mixed nuts	1 Tbsp	Fat	2.2

*Vitamin E can be stated as IUs or as the amount of alpha tocopherols. The alpha tocopherol form of Vitamin E is the most potent form. Nutrition and Supplement Facts labels report Vitamin E in IUs. If you want to convert alpha tocopherols to IUs, the conversion is 15 mg of alpha-tocopherols equals about 22 IU of natural Vitamin E and 33 IU of a synthetic source.

Calcium: Top Ten Food Sources
Daily Value = 1,000 mg
Excellent Source = 200 mg   Good Source = 100–190 mg

Food	Serving	Food Group	Amount (mg)
Milk, fat-free, calcium-fortified	1 cup	Milk	500
Milk, fat-free and 1% fat	1 cup	Milk	300
Soy beverage, calcium-fortified	1 cup	Milk	368
Buttermilk (nonfat)	1 cup	Milk	285
Yogurt	1 cup	Milk	250–350
Cheese, hard	1 oz	Meat	175–250
Cheese, hard, part skim	1 oz	Meat	175–250
Custard or pudding, homemade	1/2 cup	Sweet	200–250
Salmon, canned with bones	3 oz	Meat	180–210
Greens: collards, kale, spinach, turnip	1/2 cup	Vegetable	90–180

Folate: Top Ten Food Sources
Daily Value = 400 mcg*
Excellent Source = 80 mcg   Good Source = 40–76 mcg

Food	Serving	Food Group	Amount (mcg)
Liver, chicken, cooked	3 oz	Meat	650
Cereals, dry, fortified	1/2 cup	Starch	100–300
Beans: lentils, kidney, black, or white	1/2 cup	Starch	120–180
Asparagus	1/2 cup	Vegetable	120
Spinach	1/2 cup	Vegetable	112
Lettuce, romaine	1 cup	Vegetable	80
Peas: black-eyed, split, green	1/2 cup	Starch	50–80
Vegetables: artichoke, beets, brussels sprouts, collards, and turnip greens	1/2 cup	Vegetable	50–65
Pasta, fortified	1/2 cup	Starch	50
Orange juice	1/2 cup	Fruit	30

*The FDA now requires that companies fortify many grain products, such as dry cereals and pasta, with folic acid. When fortified, they are often good sources of it. Women of child-bearing age should make sure they get enough folic acid to prevent neural tube defects in children.

Iron: Top Ten Food Sources
Daily Value = 18 mg
Excellent Source = 3.6 mg   Good Source = 1.8–3.4 mg

Food	Serving	Food Group	Amount (mg)
Clams, canned, drained	3 oz	Meat	24
Cereals, dry, fortified	1 oz	Starch	2–20
Oysters, cooked	3 oz	Meat	9
Soybeans, boiled	1/2 cup	Meat	5
Spinach	1/2 cup	Vegetable	4
White beans, cannelli, canned	1/2 cup	Starch	4
Shrimp, cooked	3 oz	Meat	3
Beef, bottom round, lean	3 oz	Meat	3
Chickpeas, canned	1/2 cup	Starch	2
Apricots	8 halves	Fruit	2

Magnesium: Top Ten Food Sources
Daily Value = 400 mg
Excellent Source = 80 mg   Good Source = 40–76 mg

Food	Serving	Food Group	Amount (mg)
Fish, white type	3 oz	Meat	40–90
Oysters, cooked	3 oz	Meat	40–90
Wheat germ	3 Tbsp	Starch	57
Greens: beet, collard, spinach, swiss chard	1/2 cup	Vegetable	57
Beans: black-eyed peas, lima, and navy	1/2 cup	Starch	50
Millet, cooked	1/2 cup	Starch	50
Peanut butter	2 Tbsp	Fat	50
Okra	1/2 cup	Vegetable	46
Yogurt, plain, nonfat	1 cup	Milk	43
Nuts: brazil, cashews, hazel	1 Tbsp	Fat	20

Potassium: Top Ten Food Sources
Daily Value = 3,500 mg
Excellent Source = 700 mg   Good Source = 350–665 mg

Food	Serving	Food Group	Amount (mg)
Beet greens	1/2 cup	Vegetable	655
White beans, cannellini	1/2 cup	Starch	595
Yogurt, nonfat plain	1 cup	Milk	579
Clams, canned	3 oz	Meat	534
Halibut, cooked	3 oz	Meat	490
Winter squash	1/2 cup	Starch	448
Spinach, cooked	1/2 cup	Vegetable	419
Tomato sauce	1/2 cup	Vegetable	405
Sweet potato, cooked	1/2 cup	Starch	375
Potato, cooked	1/2 cup	Starch	239

Dietary Supplements and Diabetes

Research shows that people with diabetes are more likely to take dietary supplements than the general public. Good quality research, however, is still very limited on dietary supplements and whether some people with diabetes would benefit from certain vitamins, minerals, and nutrients.

According to the Diabetes Supplement Health and Education Act (DSHEA), dietary supplements don't require FDA approval prior to marketing. This lack of approval leads to the marketing of many ineffective products and many unfounded product claims. A number of dietary supplements are marketed to people with diabetes. If you choose to use dietary supplements, make sure you have good scientific reason to use them and make sure you buy high-quality supplements. Read *Before You Buy* (page 77).

Below are a few of the dietary supplements that show some promise for people with diabetes in animal and human studies. Keep in mind that most of these still require more research to verify those claims. At this time, the ADA does not recommend the use of dietary supplements for most people.

Antioxidants

Nutrition experts used to believe that people with diabetes might need more antioxidants—that is, vitamins E, C, and A (as beta carotene) and other carotenoids and selenium—because diabetes is a state of oxidative stress. Oxidative stress is known to create free-radicals that may damage various tissues in the body. Some large research trials have demonstrated that the use of antioxidants didn't show a benefit. In fact, there was concern that high doses, particularly of vitamin E, might cause health problems.

This doesn't mean that you shouldn't get the amount of these nutrients suggested by the Dietary References Intakes for your age and gender. It does mean that taking these in greater volume was not found to be beneficial.

Alpha-Lipoic Acid (ALA)

ALA, an antioxidant normally made in the liver, circulates in the body in small amounts. Foods also contain only small amounts of ALA. Some studies have shown that, in people with type 2 diabetes, ALA may help the muscles use glucose more efficiently and may make tissues more sensitive to the insulin made by the body. Some studies have also found ALA to lessen the pain of diabetes nerve disease (neuropathy).

Chromium

Chromium is an essential trace mineral that the body needs to maintain normal blood glucose levels. Chromium is found in small amounts in foods like egg yolks, whole grains, and green vegetables. Chromium, in the form of chromium picolinate, may help lower blood glucose levels and improve blood lipids in people with type 2 diabetes who may be chromium-deficient; however, the research remains mixed. Chromium supplements are generally not recommended for people with diabetes at this time.

Cinnamon (the spice)

The active ingredient in cinnamon, hydroxychalcone, is thought to enhance the effectiveness of insulin and lower blood glucose. Several small studies have shown that significant amounts of cinnamon consumed per day can lower blood glucose levels; however, other research has shown no benefit. A 2008 report that analyzed a number of the studies together (meta-analysis) showed no significant benefits of cinnamon on glucose or lipid levels.

Fenugreek

Fenugreek is a legume (bean) found in India, North America, and the Mediterranean. It is used in Indian cooking and has been used for centuries as a remedy for high blood glucose levels. Like other legumes, it's high in fiber and may lower blood glucose levels by slowing the rate at which foods with carbohydrate are broken down. It may also help the body make better use of glucose. Studies with fenugreek have been done in people with type 1 and type 2 diabetes but have not generally proven its effectiveness.

Garlic

Garlic, a member of the lily family, is a common ingredient in cooking. As a dietary supplement it has been studied for several benefits, including antioxidant effects, lowering blood glucose by increasing the release of insulin, lowering blood pressure, and improving blood lipids. So far, the research on garlic's benefits for people with diabetes is inconclusive.

American Ginseng

American ginseng is one of several species of ginseng plants, and most of the positive diabetes-related research about ginseng is with the American variety. The main benefit found in animal and human studies is that ginseng lowers blood glucose, possibly by slowing the breakdown of carbohydrate.

Magnesium

Magnesium is a mineral involved in the proper breakdown of carbohydrate and in insulin action. Low levels of magnesium in humans have been associated with higher blood glucose levels and insulin resistance in adults. According to a study published in *Diabetes Care,* obese children have lower levels of magnesium than children with normal weights. The research on providing magnesium as a dietary supplement to improve blood glucose is mixed. American adults and children don't get enough magnesium. Increase the amount of magnesium you eat by choosing more of the high-magnesium foods noted in the table on page 71.

Omega-3 Fatty Acids

The benefits of omega-3 fatty acids are related to preventing and managing heart and blood vessel disease. Studies show that omega-3 acids reduce triglycerides and protect blood vessels. They may also play a role in relieving depression. There are both fish and plant sources of omega-3 fats. Certain fish, including tuna, salmon, mackerel, and sardines, contain these fats. The non-animal sources are walnuts, flaxseeds, canola, soybeans, and olive oil. You can also find eggs that contain more omega-3 fats. ADA recommends eating two or more servings of prepared fish each week to gain the various health benefits. The American Heart Association published a similar recommendation for heart protection, but did suggest that people with heart disease and/or high triglycerides may want to take a fish oil supplement in consultation with their health care provider. Learn more about omega-3 fats in the Fats chapter.

Vanadium

Vanadium is a nutrient that may act like insulin and may help make insulin receptors better able to use glucose. Several small human studies with vanadium showed that vanadium decreased fasting blood glucose and A1C levels and improved insulin sensitivity.

Vitamin D

Vitamin D is a fat-soluble vitamin. Its chief role is to promote the absorption of calcium and phosphorus, which are essential nutrients for the health of your bones, teeth, and muscles. It's also called the "sunshine vitamin" because it's produced in your body when ultraviolet rays from

● **QUICK TIP**

Look for ways to incorporate more vitamin D in foods and consider getting a few minutes of sun each day before you put on sunscreen. You may want to talk to your health care provider about getting more vitamin D with a supplement. Often calcium and vitamin D are combined in one supplement.

sunlight strike your skin and trigger vitamin D synthesis. Vitamin D obtained from sun exposure, food, and supplements is biologically inactive and must undergo two chemical reactions in the body to activate it. The first occurs in your liver and converts vitamin D to 25-hydroxyvitamin D [25(OH)D], also known as calcidiol. The second occurs primarily in your kidney and forms the physiologically active 1,25-dihydroxyvitamin D [1,25(OH)2D], also known as calcitriol.

There's growing interest in vitamin D because larger amounts have shown positive effects on longevity, heart disease, memory loss, depression, obesity, and cancer. Research has shown that children with insufficient vitamin D intake may be at a higher risk of type 1 diabetes. The American Academy of Pediatrics is now recommending 400 IU/day of vitamin D for infants, children, and adolescents, double the previous recommendations. It has also been shown that a deficit of vitamin D damages the insulin-making beta cells and impairs the output of insulin in people with type 2 diabetes, which increases insulin resistance.

As research shows a greater need for vitamin D, peoples' intake has dwindled with the use of sunscreen to block ultraviolet rays, along with a lack of milk consumption. Currently, there is an ongoing expert panel at the Institute of Medicine looking at raising the 1997 DRIs for both calcium and vitamin D.

Learn More

Office of Dietary Supplements at National Institutes of Health, http://ods.od.nih.gov/
Office of Nutritional Products, Labeling, and Dietary Supplements, http://vm.cfsan.fda.gov/~dms/supplmnt.html

Before You Buy

Tips to consider before you purchase and start taking any dietary supplements:

- Tell your health care providers about the dietary supplements you take or ask them about supplements you want to take. They might advise you not to take a particular supplement, or they might ask you to stop taking one before surgery or another medical procedure.
- Be aware that even the recommended dose of a supplement can occasionally cause side effects. Some supplements also interact with other supplements or prescribed medicines, so be sure to discuss the supplements you use with your health care provider.
- If you believe you have some nutrition gaps, start with a multivitamin and mineral supplement. In addition to eating a wide variety of healthy foods, this approach gives you an insurance policy against your potential nutrition gaps.
- Continue to take your blood glucose–lowering medicines. If you think a dietary supplement may be making your blood glucose levels too low, talk to your health care provider about decreasing your doses of either your medicines or the supplement.
- Keep in mind that your prescription blood glucose–lowering medicines, taken in the correct doses, are more likely to reliably lower your blood glucose compared with less well-researched dietary supplements.
- Spend your money wisely. Try supplements that have been extensively researched with the greatest number of positive results.
- Use the Supplement Facts label required on all dietary supplements, to learn more about the product before you buy it.
- Start one supplement at a time. Take it in the recommended dose, and take it for a month to see if it does what it promises.
- Buy quality products that are made in the United States. Look for USP, NF, TruLabel, or Consumer Labs on the label. Buy products that have an expiration date.

Chapter 8

Blood Pressure Control: Sodium, Potassium, and More

What You'll Learn:

- the differences between salt and sodium
- recommendations for sodium intake
- the connection between high blood pressure and diabetes
- the health risks of high blood pressure
- the ADA target goal for blood pressure
- ways to decrease the amount of salt and sodium you eat
- lifestyle changes to lower high blood pressure

How Much Sodium Do Americans Eat?

Sodium and salt are different. Salt is sodium chloride, which is about 40% sodium and 60% chloride. One quarter of a teaspoon of salt contains 575 milligrams (mg) of sodium. Most Americans eat too much sodium—between 4,000 and 6,000 mg a day. Many people think that salt adds the largest amount of sodium to the American diet, but this is not true. More than half of the sodium is from the salt- and sodium-containing ingredients in manufactured and restaurant foods. Salt adds about 10–15%, and then another 10–15% comes from the natural sodium in foods.

How Much Sodium (and Potassium) Do You Need?

The answer concerning how much sodium you need appears to be creeping downward. The current Daily Value used for Nutrition Facts is 2,400 mg and the current DRI is 2,300 mg for healthy people. It's 1,500 mg for people with high blood pressure, African-American adults, and adults age 50+. Data from more current research studies show that a sodium intake of 1,500 mg per day is even better for nearly 70% of the population, including children, but especially for adults over 45.

● QUICK TIP

Studies show that the impact of lowering sodium intake and getting your fill of fruits, vegetables, and dairy foods has an additive effect on lowering blood pressure.

The BIG problem is with our current eating style. Keeping your intake of sodium small is very difficult to achieve if you eat even small amounts of processed and restaurant foods. Luckily, there's currently a major push coming from the government to food manufacturers and restaurants to lower the sodium counts of their foods. Research shows that the best approach is to slowly lower the sodium counts and allow consumers time to readjust their palates.

Due to the high intake of sodium on blood pressure, recommendations now suggest people eat more potassium-rich foods like fruits, vegetables, and low-fat dairy foods. Extra potassium can blunt the impact of too much sodium, reduce the risk of developing kidney stones, and may decrease bone loss associated with aging. Potassium plays a role in the proper functioning of the heart and helps maintain good blood pressure. The magic number is at least 4,700 mg of potassium each day.

Diabetes and High Blood Pressure

Nearly three-quarters of adults with diabetes have blood pressure that is greater than or equal to the ADA goal of 130/80 mmHg and/or take high blood pressure medication. Heart disease and stroke, often associated with high blood pressure, account for nearly two-thirds of deaths in people with diabetes. African Americans and people who are overweight are more likely to have high blood pressure. In addition, many people who have insulin resistance and/or pre-diabetes and are on the road to developing type 2 diabetes also have high blood pressure.

High blood pressure over the years can lead to many health problems. It can cause damage to your large blood vessels and can result in heart disease or stroke. It can also damage your body's small blood vessels and result in diabetic eye, nerve, and kidney disease.

Lifestyle Changes to Lower Blood Pressure

There are many changes you can make in your lifestyle to get and keep your blood pressure on target and prevent damage to your large and small blood vessels. Many of these steps are the same ones discussed throughout this book because they're simply part of healthy eating. These changes may help some people lower their blood pressure with or without medication in the short or long term. Most people who

> ● QUICK TIP
>
> What's most important
> for your long-term
> health is to get and
> keep your blood
> pressure in the target
> range: less than
> 130/80 mmHg.

have high blood pressure still need blood pressure medication and you may need to add more medications over time to control it. Consider these life-style changes additive. What's most important for your long-term health is for you to get and keep your blood pressure in the target range: less than 130/80 mmHg.

Step #1: Eat Less Sodium and Shake Less Salt

Many research studies have shown that lowering your sodium intake can help you lower both the systolic (the top number) and the diastolic (the lower number) portions of your blood pressure reading. The best-known study to date is the DASH (Dietary Approaches to Stop Hypertension) study, which reported the effects of three different eating plans on blood pressure. The lowest-sodium group ate 1,500 mg a day, the intermediate group ate 2,400 mg a day, and the high-sodium group ate 3,600 mg a day.

People on the lowest-sodium eating plan who also ate healthy amounts of grains, low-fat, high-calcium dairy foods (3 servings/day), fruits (4–6 servings/day), and vegetables (3–6 servings/day) lowered their blood pressure the most. Amazingly, the effect of the healthy eating plan was evident within one week and had the greatest effect on lowering blood pressure in just two weeks! To continue to have lower blood pressure, you need to continue to follow a lower-sodium eating plan. For some people, the lower-sodium plan reduced their blood pressure as much as a blood pressure medicine would.

Some people—especially those who are over age 50, who are African American, or who have high blood pressure or diabetes—are known to be "salt sensitive." In other words, they are especially sensitive to the blood pressure–raising effects of sodium and salt. The good news is that salt-sensitive people have a better response to eating less sodium and salt than people who aren't salt sensitive. The only way to tell if you are salt sensitive is to see if your blood pressure decreases when you consume a lower-sodium eating plan.

Tips to Reduce the Sodium in Processed and Restaurant Foods

- Review the sodium count on the Nutrition Facts labels. Foods that have less than 140 mg per serving are low in sodium.
- Use more unprocessed fresh foods. Buy fresh fruits and vegetables.
- Limit your use of ready-to-eat and processed foods, such as canned soup, cold cuts, cereals, hot dogs, frozen entrées, salad dressings, and packaged mixes.
- Choose fish, chicken, and meats that are not processed, smoked, or prepared with sauces or seasonings.
- Choose snack foods and crackers that contain less than 150–200 mg of sodium for each serving.
- Choose frozen meals or fast foods that contain less than 600–800 mg of sodium for each serving.
- Choose natural cheeses such as mozzarella or cheddar rather than processed cheeses.
- Limit condiments, such as soy or teriyaki sauce, olives, pickles, and low-fat salad dressing.
- Make your own salad dressings with a healthy oil, such as corn, safflower, canola, or soybean oil, or a blend of canola and soybean oil that's low in saturated fat. Add vinegar, mustard, fruit or vegetable juice, fresh ground pepper, garlic, and herbs.
- Limit how often you eat restaurant foods. When you do eat restaurant meals, avoid the special sauces on sandwiches and the pickles, use oil and vinegar rather than prepared salad dressing, and have fresh salads or cooked vegetables.

Tips to Use Less Salt

- Don't use salt in cooking. Get creative with herbs, spices, and seasoning. Most of them are very low in sodium.
- Don't add salt to rice, pasta, or hot cereals, as the box suggests, when you cook them.
- Take the salt off the table.

#2: Eat More Potassium

Increase your potassium intake from fruits and vegetables. Choose from high-potassium vegetables, such as broccoli, spinach, white potatoes, sweet potatoes, or winter squash. Select from high potassium fruits, such as oranges, cantaloupe, bananas, and apricots.

#3: Eat More Low-fat Dairy Foods

Low-fat dairy foods can help lower blood pressure because of their potassium and calcium content. It's known that people don't get enough of either nutrient. Eat or drink the number of servings of low-fat or fat-free dairy foods you need each day. Read more about calcium and dairy foods in chapter 12.

#4: Sip Moderate Amounts of Alcohol Only

A moderate amount of alcohol—one drink a day for women and two drinks a day for men—doesn't raise blood pressure; however, having more than three drinks a day has been shown to raise blood pressure in men and women. Read more about alcohol in chapter 17.

#5: Be Physically Active Just about Every Day

Being physically active nearly every day is an important step in preventing or controlling high blood pressure, and it can help you reduce your risk of heart disease. Being physically active can also assist with weight loss and help you keep the pounds off.

#6: Lose a Few Pounds

Research shows that losing even 10 pounds can lower blood pressure. Weight loss has the greatest effect on blood pressure in people who are overweight and already have high blood pressure.

#7: Do Not Smoke or, If You Do, Quit

Smoking cigarettes has been shown to injure blood vessel walls and speed up the process of hardening of the arteries. Even though smoking doesn't directly cause high blood pressure, it's not healthy for anyone, especially if you have high blood pressure.

#8: Diagnose and Treat Sleep Apnea

Sleep apnea, which nearly half of people with diabetes have been shown to have, can lead to high blood pressure as well as type 2 diabetes. Unfortunately, sleep apnea often goes undetected and untreated way too often. If you have signs and symptoms of sleep apnea, such as snoring, being tired during the day, and irregular breathing during sleep, discuss a sleep study with your health care provider. Treatments for sleep apnea are available.

As you can see, there are many lifestyle changes to make to get or keep your blood pressure in control. Try a few steps at a time. Get the feeling of success under your belt and then try a few more. Tackle the steps that are easiest for you to accomplish first.

SECTION 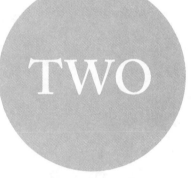 TWO

Foods by Group

Chapter 9

Starches

What You'll Learn:

- the foods in the starch food group and their nutrition assets
- healthy eating goals for the starch food group
- questions to ask yourself to get to know your current eating habits
- number of servings of starches to eat based on your calorie needs
- tips to help you buy, prepare, and eat more healthy starches filled with whole grains, dietary fiber, and other nutrients
- the serving sizes and nutrition numbers for starches

Foods in the Starch Group

Starches include all foods made from grains, such as bread, hot and dry cereal, rice, pasta, and crackers. The group also contains starchy vegetables like potatoes, corn, peas, and legumes (beans, peas, and lentils).

In general, starches provide a ready source of energy because they contain mainly carbohydrate. They are also good sources of some B vitamins, magnesium, copper, iron, selenium, and dietary fiber (if they are whole grain). The orange-colored starches, such as sweet potatoes, winter (butternut) squash, and pumpkin are great sources of carotenoids (vitamin A). White potatoes are loaded with vitamin C. White potatoes, sweet potatoes, and winter squash are full of potassium.

> ● **QUICK TIP**
>
> Eat at least half of your starch servings from whole-grain choices each day.

Green Light on Whole Grains

Studies show that eating more whole grains and dietary fiber can have both immediate and long-term health benefits. In the short term, eating more whole grains and fiber can keep your bowels regular and help you have softer bowel movements that pass from your body more easily. Whole grains and dietary fiber provide a greater feeling of fullness and may also help you lose weight and keep it off. In the long term, diets that contain whole grains have been shown to decrease the risk for heart disease, type 2 diabetes, and colon cancer.

Whole grains contain the entire grain kernel—the bran, germ, and endosperm. If the kernel has been cracked, crushed, or flaked during processing, it must retain the same relative amounts of the bran, germ, and endosperm to be called "whole grain." Examples of whole grains are whole-wheat flour, oatmeal, corn (as cornmeal), quinoa, and brown wild rice, barley, and millet.

The refining process removes most of the bran and some of the germ; it also gives the grains a finer texture and helps them last longer on the supermarket shelf. Removing the bran and germ removes the dietary fiber, along with some of the vitamins, minerals, and micronutrients.

Keep in mind that most refined grains in foods today are enriched. This means that certain B vitamins, such as thiamin, riboflavin, niacin, folic acid, and iron, are added back after processing. In fact, a federal law now requires enriched grains to be fortified with folic acid to help prevent neural tube birth defects. Fiber, however, is not added back to enriched grains. One serving of whole grain equals 16 grams of whole-grain ingredients.

● **QUICK TIP**

Don't look for whole grains on the Nutrition Facts label. They're not listed. Some manufacturers choose to put a stamp on their products telling how much whole grain is contained in a serving. Learn more about whole grains at www.wholegrainscouncil.org or www.wheatfoods.org.

Whole Grains vs. Fiber

What's the difference between whole grains and fiber? Foods made with or containing whole grains contain some fiber. But fiber is in more foods than just whole grains and there's more nutrition benefit to whole grains than just dietary fiber. Fiber is also found in fruits; starchy vegetables, such as corn and peas; legumes, such as beans, peas, and lentils; and in nonstarchy vegetables, such as broccoli, green beans, and carrots. Learn more about fiber on page 31.

Mixed Up with Fat and Sugar

Whole grains, beans, and starchy vegetables can be very healthy or they can be loaded with fat and sugar. Sometimes fat is added before we eat the food. Consider corn on the cob glistening with butter,

Healthy Potatoes?

Americans eat a lot of potatoes, and there's nothing wrong with potatoes. Unfortunately, we eat most of our potatoes as french fries and potato chips, or we eat them baked and loaded with sour cream and butter. Here is an example of how a healthy, naturally fat-free baked potato quickly becomes high in saturated fat:

1 medium (6 oz) baked potato = 160 calories,
0% calories from fat
+ 2 tsp stick margarine = 90 calories,
100% calories from fat
+ 2 Tbsp sour cream = 45 calories,
100% calories from fat

Now the baked potato has 295 calories, and 46% of those calories are from fat.

pasta covered with cheese or cream sauce, or a bagel slathered with cream cheese. Sometimes fat or sugar is added by a manufacturer or restaurant before we eat it. Consider sweetened dry cereals, packaged sweetened oatmeal, fried snack foods, and glazed donuts. In many instances, this added fat is the unhealthy saturated and trans fat type. There's room for improvement! It's a healthy eating challenge to figure out how to get and eat your starches before they get mixed up with fat and sugar.

Get to Know Yourself

If you want to change your eating habits, you need to know what and how you eat now. Ask yourself these questions about starches:

- How many starch servings do I eat on most days?
- What starches do I choose? Are they whole grains? Are they high in fiber?

- Do I eat enough whole grains (at least half of your starch servings)?
- Do the starches I choose have fat in, on, or around them?

How Many Starch Servings for You?

In chapter 6, you determined which calorie range was best for you. Find that calorie range in the chart on page 94 and then spot the number of starch servings to eat each day. It should be somewhere between 6 and 13. This might seem like a lot but because you often eat two to three starch servings in one meal, you may have to cut down. For instance, you might make a sandwich with two slices of whole-grain bread. That's two starch servings for the bread and even more if you grab a handful of chips. Let's say that you have two cups of pasta. That's six starch servings and even more if you add some garlic bread.

Get to Know Your Serving Sizes

The chart on pages 100–105 at the end of this chapter shows serving sizes for many starches you commonly eat, along with their calories, carbohydrate, fat, and fiber. One starch serving contains an average of 15 grams of carbohydrates, 3 grams of protein, and 80 calories.

In general, 1 starch serving =
- 1/2 cup of cooked cereal or starchy vegetable
- 1/3 cup grain or pasta
- 1 oz of dry cereal
- 1 oz (usually 1 slice) of bread
- 3/4–1 oz of most snack foods like pretzels and crackers

It's important to eat the correct serving size, so weigh and measure your foods occasionally to make sure you're estimating correctly. Use the same bowls and cups to help you "eyeball" the proper amount. For example, always eat your cereal out of the same bowl or serve your pasta on the same plate.

Find Your Calorie Range					
Which category fits you?	Women who… • want to lose weight • are small in size • and/or are sedentary	Women who… • are older and smaller • are larger and want to lose weight • and/or are sedentary	Women who… • are moderate to large size Men who… • are older • are small to moderate size and want to lose weight	Children Teen girls Women who… • are larger size and active Men who… • are small to moderate size and are at desired body weight	Teen boys Men who… • are active and moderate to large size
Daily calorie range	1,200–1,400	1,400–1,600	1,600–1,900	1,900–2,300	2,300–2,800
How Many Servings of Starches Do You Need Each Day?					
Starches	6	7	8	11	13

High-Fat Starches and Low-Fat Alternatives

Food	Serving	Calories	Fat (g)
Muffin	3 oz	158	4
Bagel	3 oz	178	2
Croissant	1	109	6
Bread	1 slice	65	1
Potato chips	1 oz	152	10
Potato chips, fat-free	1 oz	100	1
French fries	Small order	230	10
Baked potato	Small, 3 oz	98	0
Taco shell	1	100	6
Tortilla, corn	1	56	1
Macaroni and cheese	6 oz	250	13
Spaghetti and tomato sauce	6 oz	209	2
Refried beans	1/2 cup	136	3
Refried beans, fat-free	1/2 cup	93	0

Sample Meal Plan

The sample meal plan on page 97 gives you an idea how to fit seven starch servings into an eating plan with 1,400–1,600 calories a day. Chapter 6 provides sample plans for other calorie ranges, along with nutrition information for several plans.

Healthy Starches Challenge

To choose healthier starches you'll face a few challenges:

1. choosing starches with whole grains and fiber
2. adding more healthy starches to your meals, and
3. selecting starch toppings that are low in fat or fat-free.

These tips will help you be successful.

Breads

- Choose breads that say a slice contains at least 8 grams of whole grain on the package or in the ingredients list: 100%

whole wheat, whole grain [name of grain], whole wheat, stone-ground whole [wheat]. (Bread being brown in color doesn't mean it's whole grain. It may simply contain molasses.)

- Choose bread that contains at least 2 grams of fiber per serving.
- Choose a small whole-grain roll instead of a biscuit, scone, or croissant, which contain fat.

Crackers

- Choose low-fat or fat-free crackers made with whole grains instead of butter crackers made from enriched flour.
- Choose crackers with at least 2 grams of fiber per serving.

Cereals

- Pick whole-grain dry cereals made from bran that contain at least 3 to 5 grams of fiber per serving.
- Mix a few dry cereals together. Use one very high fiber cereal, like All-Bran, that contains 8 or more grams of fiber per serving and then mix in small amounts of other whole-grain cereals you enjoy. Top it off with ground flax.
- Get a few extra grams of fiber from hot cereal by opting for oatmeal or oat bran rather than cream of wheat or grits. Cook it with ground flax or wheat germ. (Skip the instant packaged cereals.)

Rice and Pasta

- Choose brown rice, wild rice, or rice that contains a mixture of several types instead of white rice.
- Opt for steamed brown rice instead of steamed or fried white rice in Chinese restaurants.
- Pick whole-wheat pasta. There are many on the market.

Other Starches

- Choose whole-grain tortillas, whole-grain pizza crust, muffins, and hot dog or hamburger buns.
- If you don't buy a whole-grain product, at least make sure you choose a product with enriched flour. Enriched products have had various vitamins and minerals added back in the manufacturing process.
- Learn to prepare healthy whole grains—barley, bulgur, corn, millet, oats, quinoa, wheatberries, and whole-wheat couscous. Whole grains are becoming more widely available in supermarkets and you can search the Internet for tasty recipes.

One-Day Meal Plan: 1,400–1,600 Calories

BREAKFAST

1/2 whole grain bagel (2 oz) with	**2 starches**
1 1/2 Tbsp light cream cheese	1 fat
3/4 cup blueberries with	1 fruit
1/3 cup plain fat-free yogurt	1/2 milk

LUNCH

Tuna salad made with	
2 oz tuna (1/2 cup), water-packed	2 oz meat
1 Tbsp light mayonnaise	1 fat
2 Tbsp diced celery	1 vegetable
1 Tbsp diced onions	
Tomato slices	
2 slices whole-wheat bread	**2 starches**
1 cup raw or blanched broccoli	1 vegetable
1 cup fat-free milk	1 milk
1/2 large apple	1 fruit

DINNER

3 oz grilled salmon with	3 oz meat
lemon and herbs	free food
Stir-fried vegetables with	
1/4 cup onions, cooked	2 vegetables
1/2 cup snow peas, cooked	
1/2 cup red peppers, cooked	
2 tsp canola oil	2 fats
1 cup brown rice	**3 starches**

EVENING SNACK

Mix together:	
1/2 cup crushed canned pineapple (packed in own juice)	1 fruit
1/3 cup plain fat-free yogurt	1/2 milk
1/8 cup chopped pecans	2 fats

Easy Ways to Eat More Healthy Starches

- In a meatloaf or meatball recipe, substitute whole-grain bread, bulgur, or brown rice in place of some meat.
- Add whole-wheat pasta, peas, or beans to a vegetable soup.
- Prepare a hearty bean or pea soup as a main course. Divide the leftovers into individual portions and store them in the freezer for a quick meal.
- Substitute whole-grain flour and/or cornmeal for half the flour in pancake or waffle batter and in muffins or breads.
- When you cook a whole grain, make enough for extra servings. Toss the leftovers on salad or into soups or casseroles. Mix in toasted nuts or dried fruit to make them even healthier.
- Eat whole-grain dry cereal without milk as a snack on the run or mixed with yogurt and dried fruit for a healthy snack at home.
- Toss leftover cold corn, brown rice, bulgur, or peas on a salad.
- Open a can of garbanzo beans (chickpeas) or kidney beans, and add them to a salad, tomato sauce, three-bean salad, or soup.
- Have whole-wheat pretzels or light popcorn for a snack.
- Use winter squash, acorn squash, and sweet potatoes frequently. They are loaded with vitamin A.

Use Low-Fat or Fat-Free Starch Toppers

- Spread soft or light cream cheese on bagels or toast.
- Put reduced-calorie sour cream or plain yogurt mixed with fresh or dried herbs on baked potatoes.
- Put cottage cheese in the blender to make it smooth. Mix in herbs or seasonings to top pasta or baked potatoes.
- Put a tasty mustard on baked potatoes or sandwiches.
- Mix tomato sauce with whole-grain pasta or brown rice.
- Choose a tub margarine made without trans fats.
- Use low-fat or fat-free mayonnaise on sandwiches.
- Put salsa on low-fat tortilla chips, Mexican burritos, or fajitas.

Julie's Story

Julie is 64 years old and has had type 2 diabetes for about 10 years. Julie has managed her diabetes fairly well until recently. She has gained about 15 pounds over the last year, in part because she finally quit smoking. She was also very stressed about one of her granddaughters who was ill. Her doctor was pleased that Julie quit smoking because her blood pressure decreased. However, her doctor was concerned about her weight gain, especially because her A1C has been climbing. Her last A1C reading was 9.3%, which means her blood glucose is averaging about 220 mg/dl.

Julie recently started taking a long-acting insulin at night in addition to two blood glucose–lowering pills. Her doctor suggested that she meet with a registered dietitian (RD) to help her control her weight gain and lower her blood glucose. Julie met with the RD, and they reviewed her current eating habits. The dietitian suggested that Julie eat more starches and smaller amounts of meats and fat. So, instead of some meat at breakfast, Julie will try to eat fruit, 2 starches, and a cup of fat-free milk. For her starches, Julie will eat a whole-wheat English muffin topped with light cream cheese and low-sugar jam, dry cereal, or oat bran. On occasion, she will try a whole-grain frozen waffle with two teaspoons of regular maple syrup.

At lunch, Julie will decrease the amount of meat in her sandwiches. She'll add another starch and some crunch with baked tortilla chips or potato chips or whole-wheat pretzels, or she will toss garbanzo or kidney beans on her salad.

At dinner, she will try a few new quick-to-fix recipes that have more starches—chili made with turkey sausage over a baked potato; a store-bought pizza with a whole-grain crust to which she will add broccoli, red peppers, and sliced tomatoes; or whole-grain pasta with a light, tomato-based meat sauce. This is certainly a switch for Julie, who remembers how she always looked for ways to cut down on starches.

Serving Sizes for Starches

Food	Serving Size	Calories	Carb (g)	Fat (g)	Fiber (g)
BREADS					
Bagel, plain	1/4 large	78	15.1	0.5	0.6
Biscuit, baked	1 biscuit (2 1/2" dia)	127	17.0	5.8	0.5
Bread, pumpernickel	1 slice (5" x 4" x 3/8")	80	15.2	1.0	2.1
Bread, raisin	1 slice	71	13.6	1.1	1.1
Bread, reduced-calorie wheat	2 slices	91	20.1	1.1	5.5
Bread, reduced-calorie white	2 slices	95	20.4	1.1	4.5
Bread, rye, light or dark	1 slice, thick	83	15.5	1.1	1.9
Bread, white	1 slice	67	12.4	0.9	0.6
Bread, whole-wheat	1 slice	69	12.9	1.2	1.9
Chappatti	1 small (6" across)	71	15.1	0.4	1.9
Cornbread, baked	1 1/2 ozs	113	18.5	3.0	1.0
English muffin	1/2 muffin	67	13.1	0.5	0.8
Hamburger bun or roll	1/2 small bun	60	10.6	0.9	0.5
Hot dog bun or roll	1/2 bun	61	10.8	1.1	0.6
Naan	1/4 large (8" x 2")	75	0.6	2.0	0.6

Pancake plain, frozen, reheated	1 pancake (4" dia)	82	15.7	1.2	0.6
Pita bread, white	1/2 pita	82	16.7	0.4	0.7
Roll, plain dinner	1 roll (1 oz)	85	14.3	2.1	0.9
Stuffing, bread, prepared	1/3 cup	117	14.3	5.7	1.9
Taco shells	2 medium (5" dia)	124	16.6	6.0	2.0
Tortilla, corn, ready to bake or fry	1 medium (6" dia)	52	10.7	0.7	1.5
Tortilla, flour, 10" across	1/3 tortilla	72	11.9	1.8	0.7
Tortilla, flour, 6" across	1 tortilla	112	15.4	2.8	1.1
Waffle, toaster style	1 waffle (4" dia)	96	14.6	3.3	0.5
CEREALS					
All-Bran Cereal (Kellogg)	1/2 cup	81	22.9	1.0	9.9
Bran, oat, uncooked	1/4 cup	58	15.6	1.7	3.6
Bran, 100%, wheat, unprocessed	1/2 cup	63	18.7	1.2	12.4
Cheerios	2/3 cup	83	16.6	1.4	2.0
Corn flakes	2/3 cup	76	18.1	0.2	0.7
Fiber One Bran Cereal (General Mills)	1/2 cup	59	24.3	0.8	14.4
Frosted Flakes Cereal (Kellogg)	1/2 cup	76	18.6	0.1	0.7
Granola	1/4 cup	125	19.0	4.9	1.3
Granola cereal, low-fat	1/4 cup	86	18.0	1.1	1.1

(continues)

Adapted from *Choose Your Foods: Exchange Lists for Diabetes* (American Dietetic Association and American Diabetes Association, 2008).

Serving Sizes for Starches *(continued)*

Food	Serving Size	Calories	Carb (g)	Fat (g)	Fiber (g)
Muesli	1/4 cup	74	15.1	1.1	1.5
Oatmeal, cooked	1/2 cup	73	12.6	1.2	2.0
Puffed rice cereal	1 1/2 cups	80	18.4	0.2	0.3
Puffed wheat cereal	1 1/2 cups	66	13.8	0.4	1.7
Rice krispies	3/4 cup	77	17.4	0.3	0.1
Shredded wheat, plain	1/2 cup	83	20.3	0.3	2.8
Wheaties Cereal (General Mills)	3/4 cup	80	18.2	0.7	2.3
CRACKERS/SNACKS					
Animal crackers	8 crackers	89	14.8	2.8	0.2
Crackers, round butter type	6 crackers	90	11.0	4.6	0.3
Crackers, saltines	6 crackers	77	12.8	2.0	0.5
Crackers, whole wheat, baked	5 crackers	89	13.7	3.4	2.1
Crackers, whole wheat, reduced-fat	5 triscuits	80	15.0	2.0	2.5
Crispbread	2 slices	73	16.4	0.3	3.3
Graham crackers	3 crackers (2 1/2" square)	99	18.0	2.4	0.7
Matzoh crackers, plain	3/4 oz	83	17.6	0.3	0.6

Melba toast	4 pieces (3 3/4" x 1 3/4" x 1/8")	78	15.3	0.6	1.3
Oyster crackers	20 crackers	86	14.2	2.3	0.6
Pita chips, baked	3/4 oz	86	11.8	3.1	0.4
Popcorn, microwave, 94% fat free, popped	3 cups	65	14.0	1.3	2.5
Popcorn, microwave, with butter, popped	3 cups	96	10.8	6.0	1.8
Popcorn, popped, no salt or fat added	3 cups	93	18.7	1.1	3.5
Potato chips	3/4 oz	114	11.2	7.3	0.7
Potato Chips, baked	3/4 oz	82	17.2	1.1	1.5
Potato chips, fat-free	3/4 oz	56	13.5	0.0	0.7
Pretzels, sticks or rings	3/4 oz	80	16.6	0.7	0.7
Rice cakes	2 cakes	70	14.7	0.5	0.8
Sandwich crackers, cheese filled	3 sandwiches	100	13.0	4.4	0.4
Sandwich crackers, peanut butter	3 sandwiches	102	12.3	5.0	0.6
Tortilla chips	3/4 oz	106	13.4	5.6	0.4
Tortilla chips, fat-free	3/4 oz	82	18.0	0.8	3.0
STARCHY VEGETABLES					
Cassava, cooked	1/3 cup, diced	70	16.7	0.1	0.8
Corn on cob, cooked	1/2 large ear	66	16.0	0.5	2.0

(continues)

Adapted from *Choose Your Foods: Exchange Lists for Diabetes* (American Dietetic Association and American Diabetes Association, 2008).

Serving Sizes for Starches (continued)

Food	Serving Size	Calories	Carb (g)	Fat (g)	Fiber (g)
Corn, canned, drained	1/2 cup	66	15.2	0.8	1.6
Corn, frozen cooked	1/2 cup	66	16.0	0.4	2.0
Hominy, canned, drained, rinsed	3/4 cup	90	17.8	1.1	3.1
Parsnips, fresh, cooked	1/2 cup	63	15.2	0.2	3.1
Pasta (spaghetti) sauce, traditional, meatless	1/4 cup	128	17.6	3.5	2.0
Peas, green, frozen cooked	1/2 cup	62	11.4	0.2	4.4
Plantain, ripe, cooked	1/3 cup, slices	59	15.8	0.1	1.2
Potato, baked with skin	3 ozs	79	18.0	0.1	1.9
Potato, fresh, mashed, made with milk	1/2 cup	85	19.0	0.3	1.7
Potato, white, peeled, cooked	3 ozs	73	17.0	0.1	1.5
Potatoes, french-fried, frozen, oven baked	1 cup	98	16.4	3.0	1.5
Pumpkin, canned	1 cup	83	19.8	0.7	7.1
Squash, winter, cooked	1 cup	39	8.8	0.6	2.8
Succotash (lima beans and corn), frozen	1/2 cup	79	17.0	0.8	3.5
Vegetables, mixed (corn, peas, carrots), frozen, cooked	1 cup	80	17.7	0.2	4.0

Vegetables, mixed (with pasta), frozen cooked	1 cup	80	14.7	0.2	5.0
Yams, cooked	1/2 cup	79	18.8	0.1	2.7
BEANS/PEAS/LENTILS					
Beans, baked, no pork	1/3 cup	78	17.2	0.4	4.2
Beans, black, cooked	1/2 cup	114	20.4	0.5	7.5
Beans, kidney, cooked	1/2 cup	112	20.2	0.4	5.7
Beans, lima, canned, drained	1/2 cup	99	18.0	0.3	6.0
Beans, lima, frozen cooked	1/2 cup	76	14.3	0.3	4.4
Beans, navy, cooked	1/2 cup	129	23.9	0.5	5.8
Beans, pinto, cooked	1/2 cup	122	22.3	0.6	7.7
Beans, white, cooked	1/2 cup	125	22.6	0.3	5.7
Chickpeas (garbanzo beans), cooked	1/2 cup	134	22.5	2.1	6.2
Lentils, cooked	1/2 cup	115	19.9	0.4	7.8
Peas, black-eyed (crowder), cooked	1/2 cup	100	17.9	0.5	5.6
Refried beans, canned	1/2 cup	100	17.0	0.5	6.0
Split peas, cooked	1/2 cup	116	20.7	0.4	8.1

Adapted from *Choose Your Foods: Exchange Lists for Diabetes* (American Dietetic Association and American Diabetes Association, 2008).

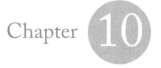
Vegetables

What You'll Learn:

- the foods in the vegetable food group and their nutrition assets
- healthy eating goals for vegetables
- a frame of reference about how many vegetables people eat now
- questions to ask yourself to get to know your current eating habits
- the number of servings of vegetables to eat based on your calorie needs
- tips to help you buy, prepare, and eat more vegetables
- the serving sizes and nutrition numbers for vegetables

Foods in the Vegetable Group

This food group includes all fresh, frozen, and canned vegetables and vegetable juices. You'll find starchy vegetables, such as corn, peas, potatoes, and winter squash, in the starch group. Consider the vegetables in this group nonstarchy.

Vegetables are an important part of your healthy eating plan. They are naturally packed with nutrition, yet low in calories. They provide lots of crunch for very few calories if they aren't fried or drowned in butter or salad dressing. Let vegetables take up about half of your plate at lunch and dinner.

The few calories in vegetables come from carbohydrate and a small amount of protein. Vegetables are good sources of fiber, vitamins, and minerals. When you vary the vegetables you eat, you get the variety of vitamins and minerals they offer. Current healthy eating recommendations suggest:

- 3 cups each week of dark green vegetables
- 2 cups a week of orange vegetables.

Nutrition Benefits of Vegetables

Different groups of vegetables have different nutrition assets:

- Dark green vegetables—which include the leafy greens, romaine, field greens, spinach, kale, broccoli, and collards— offer beta-carotene (which the body converts to vitamin A), vitamins C and E, and minerals such as calcium, folate, potassium, and magnesium.
- Broccoli, peppers (all colors), cabbage, Brussels sprouts, and tomatoes are high in vitamin C.
- Orange vegetables, such as carrots, are a top source of beta-carotene. (Many of the other healthy orange vegetables, such as sweet potatoes and winter squash, are in the starch group.)

Nutrition studies have shown the benefits of eating vegetables (these studies usually also consider the benefits of eating more fruit as well). Together, vegetables and fruit have been shown to reduce the risk for and help manage type 2 diabetes, high blood pressure, and heart disease. They also protect against certain cancers, such as mouth, stomach, and colon cancer.

Vegetables: How Much People Eat

Plain and simple, people don't eat enough vegetables. That's not surprising with all the on-the-go eating we do. Vegetables are just not plentiful in these venues. People also don't vary their vegetable choices or take advantage of the most nutritious varieties. For example, many people choose iceberg lettuce for salads instead of opting for spinach, arugula, red leaf, and/or romaine lettuce.

When you make quick-to-fix meals—perhaps a frozen chicken entrée or a package of macaroni and cheese—you may not take time to cut vegetables for a salad or to steam fresh asparagus. Some people say, "I don't buy vegetables because they turn brown before I use them. I throw out more than I eat." If you don't buy vegetables, you cannot eat them, and if you eat them, they won't go bad.

Restaurant meals and eating on the run can make getting enough vegetables even more difficult. It's just not as easy to wolf down a salad in your car as it is a burger and fries. More pizzas are topped with pepperoni and extra cheese than onions, mushrooms, and peppers. In fancy restaurants, your plate may be delivered with tiny vegetable portions because the chef is focused on the entrée—the meat, poultry, or seafood. It's easy to understand why we have trouble following Mom's advice to "eat your vegetables."

● **QUICK TIP**

People often consider vegetables a side dish, not the main course. There are many delicious ways to prepare and add vegetables to meals, so go ahead and fill your plate with them.

Just as starches and fat taste good together, so do vegetables. Vegetables are healthy, but that's before you douse lettuce greens with blue cheese dressing, cover green beans with cream of mushroom soup and fried onion rings, or order a fried onion or zucchini appetizer. Fat adds too many calories, and sometimes those calories are from unhealthy saturated fat.

Healthy Broccoli?

Here are the numbers to show how a healthy helping of broccoli quickly becomes unhealthy with added fat in the cheese sauce:

1 cup cooked broccoli = 44 calories,
0% calories from fat

+ 2 Tbsp cheese sauce = 36 calories, (4 g fat)
100% calories from fat

Now the broccoli has 80 calories, and 45% of those calories are from fat.

Get to Know Yourself

If you want to change your eating habits, learn what you eat now. Ask yourself these questions about vegetables:

- How many vegetable servings do I eat on average each day?
- What vegetables do I eat? Is it a narrow or varied list?
- Do I eat some raw vegetables every day?
- Do I buy vegetables packaged with a lot of fat and sodium?
- Do I add or prepare vegetables with fat?

How Many Servings of Vegetables Do You Need?

In chapter 6 you determined that a certain calorie range was the best for you. Find that calorie range in the chart on page 112 and then spot the number of servings of vegetables you need each day. It is somewhere between 3 and 5. This might seem like a lot of vegetables to eat, and it is probably more than you currently eat. In this chapter, you'll learn easy ways to fit in more vegetables. (If you can spare the calories, more is better and more will help you fill up on fewer calories.)

The sample meal plan on page 114 shows how to fit four servings of vegetables into your day. This plan is designed for a person who needs 1,400–1,600 calories a day. Chapter 6 provides sample plans and nutritional information for other calorie ranges.

Get to Know Your Serving Sizes

The chart on pages 120–123 at the end of this chapter shows serving sizes for many vegetables you commonly eat, along with their calories, carbohydrate, and fiber content. Each vegetable serving, on average, contains about 5 grams of carbohydrate, 2 grams of protein, and 25 calories.

In general, 1 vegetable serving =
- 1 cup of raw vegetables
- 1/2 cup of cooked vegetables.

It's important to eat the correct serving size, so you may want to weigh and measure your foods occasionally to make sure you're estimating correctly; however, if there's one place going a bit overboard won't hurt much, it's nonstarchy vegetables!

The Healthy Vegetable Challenge

Do you hide vegetables under cream sauce? Do you dunk raw vegetables in a sour cream or mayonnaise-based dip? Do you buy frozen vegetables in cream or butter sauce? Do you buy canned vegetables, which can be high in sodium? Your challenge is to find ways to prepare and eat vegetables with little added fat and sodium. Make changes one at a time. For example, if you are used to putting butter or margarine on vegetables prior to serving them, instead put the tub

Find Your Calorie Range

Which category fits you?	Women who… • want to lose weight • are small in size and/or are sedentary	Women who… • are older and smaller • are larger and want to lose weight • and/or are sedentary	Women who… • are moderate to large size Men who… • are older • are small to moderate size and want to lose weight	Children Teen girls Women who… • are larger size and active Men who… • are small to moderate size and are at desired body weight	Teen boys Men who… • are active and moderate to large size
Daily calorie range	1,200–1,400	1,400–1,600	1,600–1,900	1,900–2,300	2,300–2,800

How Many Servings of Vegetables Do You Need Each Day?

Vegetables (nonstarchy)	3	4	4	5	5

of margarine on the table and let family members choose how much they want. Or better yet, don't put the margarine on the table, and instead, slice a fresh lemon or lime into wedges to squeeze on steamed vegetables. Try sprinkling cinnamon or nutmeg in the water when you microwave carrots. These ideas add flavor without adding fat.

It's also a healthy move to keep your vegetables as low in sodium as possible. Vegetables are naturally very low in sodium, but the sodium creeps in when vegetables are canned, frozen with sauces and seasonings, or topped with commercial salad dressing. Keep the sodium content of your vegetables low by using fresh or plain frozen vegetables. If you purchase canned vegetables, opt for the no-salt-added variety.

Higher-Fat Vegetable Dishes and Lower-Fat Alternatives

Food	Serving	Calories	Fat (g)
Fried zucchini, breaded and deep-fried	1/2 cup	279	16
Sauteed zucchini with broth and sherry	1/2 cup	30	0
Green bean casserole	1/2 cup	160	11
Green beans steamed with garlic and herbs	1/2 cup	22	0
Spinach soufflé	1/2 cup	110	9
Spinach and vinegar	1/2 cup	20	0
Salad with 2 Tbsp regular blue cheese dressing	1 cup salad	191	16
Salad with 2 Tbsp fat-free blue cheese dressing	1 cup salad	57	0

One-Day Meal Plan: 1,400–1,600 Calories

BREAKFAST

1/2 whole grain bagel (2 oz) with	2 starches
1 1/2 Tbsp light cream cheese	1 fat
3/4 cup blueberries with	1 fruit
1/3 cup plain fat-free yogurt	1/2 milk

LUNCH

Tuna salad made with	
2 oz tuna (1/2 cup), water-packed	2 oz meat
1 Tbsp light mayonnaise	1 fat
2 Tbsp diced celery	**1 vegetable**
1 Tbsp diced onions	
Tomato slices	
2 slices whole-wheat bread	2 starches
1 cup raw or blanched broccoli	**1 vegetable**
1 cup fat-free milk	1 milk
1/2 large apple	1 fruit

DINNER

3 oz grilled salmon with	3 oz meat
lemon and herbs	free food
Stir-fried vegetables with	
1/4 cup onions, cooked	**2 vegetables**
1/2 cup snow peas, cooked	
1/2 cup red peppers, cooked	
2 tsp canola oil	2 fats
1 cup brown rice	3 starches

EVENING SNACK

Mix together:	
1/2 cup crushed canned pineapple (packed in own juice)	1 fruit
1/3 cup plain fat-free yogurt	1/2 milk
1/8 cup chopped pecans	2 fats

Salad and Dressing—Famous Pals

Perhaps the most famous vegetable and fat combo is salad and dressing. You select a nutrition-packed salad with dark greens, tomatoes, cucumbers, carrots, and more, which contains very few calories, mainly from carbohydrate. Then you pour on a couple of tablespoons of regular salad dressing, adding 150 calories of almost pure fat. The challenge is to keep your salads nutrient rich and the fat levels low. Limit other high-fat salad toppings, too, such as cheese, pasta or potato salad, bacon bits, or fried noodles. Dress up a salad with a few healthy toppings, such as olives, nuts, raisins (or other dried or chopped fruit), or seeds.

Salad Dressing Know-How

Your choice of salad dressings is wider than ever. In the supermarket, there are regular, reduced-fat, low-calorie, and fat-free salad dressings. Note that the terms "reduced fat" and "fat free" do not mean calorie free. These dressings still contain calories. The fat-free dressings often contain more carbohydrate in place of fat and many contain even more sodium. Check out the nutrition information for the varied types of two favorite dressings, Thousand Island and Italian.

Dressing	Calories (in 2 Tbsp)	Carbohydrate (g)	Fat (g)	Sodium (mg)
THOUSAND ISLAND				
Regular	118	5	11	276
Low-calorie	61	7	4	249
Fat-free	42	9	0.5	233
ITALIAN				
Regular	109	2	11	505
Low-calorie	56	2	6	398
Fat-free	20	4	0	430

● QUICK TIP

Another factor to consider when you choose salad dressings is the oil they are made from. Most store-bought salad dressings are made from soybean oil. This is a healthy oil that contains mainly polyunsaturated fat.

Vote for Homemade Salad Dressing

One way to make sure your salad dressings are healthier—lower in total fat, contain optimal fats, and light in sodium—is to make your own. Make up a batch, store it in a cruet or spray container, and bring it to the table instead of bottled dressings. Make it with a healthy oil—one low in saturated fat. If you like the taste, use extra virgin olive oil. If you like a lighter tasting oil, use canola, sunflower, or soybean oil. Choose from a wide variety of interesting vinegars—balsamic, raspberry, or red wine. Mustard can help emulsify (blend) the dressing. Season it with herbs and spices. Tips to make your salad and dressing healthier pals:

- Don't pre-dress salads at home.
- Use as little salad dressing as you can. (Hint: If you always find dressing at the bottom of your salad, you can use less.)
- Use the fork-and-dip technique. Lightly dip a forkful of salad into the dressing.
- If you use a creamy dressing, dilute it with a few drizzles of your preferred vinegar or lemon.

Salad Dressing Tips When Eating Out

Use these tips when you eat out:

- Order salad dressing on the side.
- Opt for olive oil and vinegar.
- Request some vinegar or lemon wedges on the side to dilute the small amount of dressing.
- In fast-food restaurants, don't use the whole packet, which amounts to 1/4 cup or 4 Tbsp. Drizzle some dressing, mix up your salad, and see if you have enough.

Eat More Raw Vegetables

An easy way to eat more vegetables is to eat them raw—a few stalks of broccoli or cauliflower, a handful of cherry or grape tomatoes, a handful of baby carrots, or sticks of zucchini. If you eat raw vegetables, you don't lose vitamins and minerals to cooking. Stock the refrigerator with a ready-to-go supply of vegetables, and have a handful for lunch, dinner, or a snack. Make enough salad at one time to last a few days or chop and store the salad extras—peppers, cucumbers, carrots, onions, and the like. Store them in an airtight plastic container. If you do not like some vegetables raw but you will eat them cooked and chilled, blanch a bunch of green beans, a head of broccoli, or a handful of snow peas. Stash them in a plastic container in the refrigerator so that they are ready to eat. To blanch vegetables, boil a small amount of water with a pinch of salt and steam the vegetables for 2–3 minutes. Vegetables should be slightly soft but still crisp. Remove the pot from the stove or microwave and place the vegetables in ice water to stop the cooking process.

Tips for Buying, Preparing, and Eating More Vegetables

- Vary your vegetables. The greater the variety, the greater the mix of vitamins, minerals, and other nutrients you eat.
- Take advantage of all the ready-to-eat or easy-to-fix vegetables in the supermarket—salad in bags or boxes, baby carrots, grape and cherry tomatoes, precut celery and carrot sticks, sliced mushrooms, and bags of precut vegetable medleys ready to steam.
- Keep a bag of precut carrots around. Have a handful as a snack, pack them with lunch, add them to stew, or microwave them for a quick dish.
- Keep some frozen and low-sodium canned vegetables on hand so that you always have vegetables ready to eat.
- Use a variety of greens in salads. Use a mix of several greens—romaine, mixed field greens, arugula, or spinach. Dice in some red cabbage for color and nutrition. Choose bags of greens that combine several types.

(continues)

Tips for Buying, Preparing, and Eating More Vegetables
(continued)

- Don't buy vegetables in butter or flavor sauces.
- Make double and triple portions. Eat a serving one day and have another one ready to go for the next.
- Blanch (quick cook and chill) a head of broccoli or cauliflower, break it into pieces, place it in a plastic container, and have a ready supply for the week, hot or cold.
- Microwave or sauté onions, peppers, and mushrooms to add more vegetables to a tomato sauce or top a frozen pizza.
- Enjoy baby carrots, celery sticks, and slices of red pepper dipped in a yogurt-based dip or reduced-calorie creamy salad dressing for a low-calorie snack.
- Make a big salad to last a few days; store it in a plastic container.
- Remember, almost anything healthy can top a salad—green peas, garbanzo beans, green beans, extra bulgur, quinoa, brown rice, raisins, pineapple, dried apricots, or mandarin oranges.
- Add vegetables to sandwiches—not just the old routine lettuce and sliced tomato. Try alfalfa sprouts or slices of red onion, cucumbers, yellow squash, zucchini, or red peppers. Use healthy avocado slices instead of mayonnaise to moisten the bread.
- Add vegetables to an omelet or scrambled eggs. Sauté onions, peppers, mushrooms, and tomatoes and add some fresh herbs.
- In a tomato sauce, cut the amount of meat you use to half of the recipe and add more vegetables—onions, peppers, mushrooms, eggplant, zucchini, or others.
- Use pureed cooked vegetables such as potatoes to thicken stews, soups, and gravies. These add flavor, nutrients, and texture.

Brent's Story

Brent is 25 years old. He has had type 1 diabetes for seven years, and he takes insulin four times a day. He tries to regulate his blood glucose tightly because he wants to prevent diabetes complications, especially losing his eyesight. He is physically active with his company's softball team and works out in a gym three times a week.

Brent eats 2,500 to 3,000 calories a day to keep his weight between 177 and 180 pounds. He recently read that people should eat at least five servings of fruit and vegetables a day. When he thinks about what he eats on an average day, he realizes that he only eats, at best, two to three vegetable servings a day—lettuce and tomato on a hamburger at lunch, a salad, or maybe packaged, frozen spinach soufflé or broccoli with cheese sauce at dinner. During a recent visit with a dietitian, he set four to five servings of vegetables and fruits a day as a nutrition goal.

Brent and the RD strategized ways to fit more vegetables in each day. When Brent takes lunch to work, he will put some slices of cucumber and alfalfa sprouts on his sandwiches and take baby carrots or grape tomatoes to eat along with his sandwich. When he eats in a restaurant or cafeteria, he'll request extra lettuce, tomato, and onion on a sandwich and make a salad from the salad bar or have a hot vegetable. He will try to keep frozen vegetables in the freezer and include a double helping of vegetables at dinner. To add flavor to steamed vegetables, he will use fresh lemon or lime and only a small amount of butter. When he has pizza for dinner, he will hold the extra cheese and ground meat and request sliced tomato, onions, peppers, and mushrooms instead. He likes vegetable toppings; they're just not the usual fare when he orders pizza with friends.

To chart his progress, Brent agreed to make a note in his electronic calendar of how many servings of vegetables he eats on Monday and Thursday of each week for four weeks.

Serving Sizes for Vegetables

Food	Serving Size	Calories	Carb (g)	Fiber (g)
VEGETABLES				
Amaranth leaves (Chinese spinach), cooked	1/2 cup	14	2.7	1.2
Artichoke hearts, canned, drained	1 artichoke	15	3.0	0.5
Artichoke, cooked	1/2 artichoke	30	7.3	0.5
Asparagus, frozen cooked	1/2 cup	25	4.4	1.4
Baby corn, cocktail type, canned, drained	1/2 cup	20	5.0	2.0
Bamboo shoots, canned, drained	1/2 cup	12	2.1	0.9
Bean sprouts, fresh, cooked	1/2 cup	13	2.6	0.5
Beans, canned, drained (green, wax)	1/2 cup	14	3.1	1.3
Beans, green, fresh, cooked	1/2 cup	22	4.9	2.0
Beets, canned, drained	1/2 cup	26	6.1	1.4
Bitter melon gourd (Asian, balsam), cooked	1/2 cup (1/2" pieces)	12	2.7	1.2
Bok choy (Chinese white cabbage or pak-choy)	1 cup, shredded	9	1.5	0.7
Borscht (beet soup)	1/2 cup	39	4.1	0.9
Bottle (hairy) gourd (upo, lauki), cooked	1/2 cup, mashed	12	2.6	1.3
Broccoli, fresh cooked	1/2 cup	22	4.0	2.3

Brussels sprouts, frozen cooked	1/2 cup	33	6.5	3.3
Cabbage, fresh cooked	1/2 cup	17	3.3	1.7
Carrots, fresh cooked	1/2 cup	35	8.2	2.6
Carrots, fresh, raw	1 cup, strips or slices	50	11.7	3.7
Cauliflower, fresh, raw	1 cup	25	5.2	2.5
Cauliflower, frozen cooked	1/2 cup	17	3.4	2.4
Celery, fresh, raw	1 cup, strips	17	3.7	1.7
Chard, swiss, cooked	1/2 cup	18	3.6	1.8
Chayote squash (mirliton, sayote), cooked	1/2 cup	19	4.1	2.2
Coleslaw mix	1 cup	17	3.3	1.5
Collard greens, fresh cooked	1/2 cup	26	5.8	2.7
Cucumber, with peel	1 cup	16	3.8	0.5
Eggplant, fresh cooked	1/2 cup (1" cubes)	17	4.3	1.2
Green (spring) onions	1 cup	32	7.3	2.6
Hearts of palm, canned, not drained	1/2 cup	20	3.4	1.8
Jicama (yambean, singkamas), cooked	1/2 cup, cubes	30	6.9	3.1
Kale, fresh, cooked	1/2 cup	18	3.7	1.3

(continues)

Adapted from Choose Your Foods: Exchange Lists for Diabetes (American Dietetic Association and American Diabetes Association, 2008).

Serving Sizes for Vegetables *(continued)*

Food	Serving Size	Calories	Carb (g)	Fiber (g)
Kohlrabi, fresh cooked	1/2 cup	24	5.5	0.9
Leeks, fresh cooked	1/2 cup	16	4.0	0.5
Luffa (Chinese okra), angled, cooked	1/2 cup	20	4.0	2.0
Mixed vegetables, (no corn, peas, pasta)	1/2 cup	20	3.3	1.3
Mung bean sprouts, seed attached, cooked	1/2 cup	13	2.6	0.5
Mushrooms, fresh	1 cup	15	2.3	0.7
Mustard greens, fresh cooked	1/2 cup	10	1.5	1.4
Okra, frozen cooked	1/2 cup	34	5.3	2.6
Onions, fresh	1 cup	67	16.2	2.2
Onions, fresh cooked	1/2 cup	46	10.7	1.5
Oriental radish (daikon, labanos), raw	1 cup	21	4.8	1.9
Pea pods (snow peas), fresh cooked	1/2 cup	34	5.6	2.2
Peas, sugar snap, frozen uncooked	1/2 cup	30	5.2	1.9
Pepper, green bell, raw	1 cup, slices	18	4.3	1.6
Pepper, red, fresh cooked	1/2 cup	19	4.6	0.8
Peppers, hot chili, green, canned	1/2 cup	25	3.3	3.3

Radishes	1 cup	20	4.2	1.9
Rutabaga, fresh, cooked	1/2 cup, cubes	33	7.4	1.5
Sauerkraut, canned, rinsed, drained	1/2 cup	23	5.1	3.0
Soybean sprouts, seed attached, cooked	1/2 cup	38	3.1	0.4
Spinach, canned, drained	1/2 cup	25	3.6	2.6
Squash, summer, fresh cooked	1/2 cup	18	3.9	1.3
Squash, summer, raw	1 cup	18	3.8	1.2
Tomato juice	1/2 cup	21	5.2	0.5
Tomato sauce	1/2 cup	37	8.8	1.7
Tomato, raw	1 cup	32	7.1	2.2
Tomatoes, canned, regular	1/2 cup	24	5.5	1.3
Turnip greens, fresh cooked	1/2 cup	14	3.1	2.5
Turnips, fresh cooked	1/2 cup, diced	17	3.9	1.6
Vegetable juice	1/2 cup	25	5.5	0.5
Water chestnuts, canned, drained	1/2 cup	40	8.9	2.7
Yard-long beans, fresh cooked	1/2 cup, slices	24	4.8	1.9
Zucchini, fresh cooked	1/2 cup, slices	14	3.5	1.3
Zucchini, raw	1 cup, slices	18	3.8	1.2

Adapted from *Choose Your Foods: Exchange Lists for Diabetes* (American Dietetic Association and American Diabetes Association, 2008).

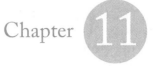
Fruits

What You'll Learn:

- the foods in the fruit food group and their nutrition assets
- healthy eating goals for the fruit group
- a frame of reference about how much fruit people eat
- questions to ask yourself to get to know your current habits
- the number of servings of fruits to eat based on your calorie needs
- tips for buying, preparing, and eating more fruits
- the serving sizes and nutrition numbers for fruits

Foods in the Fruit Group

This group includes all fresh, frozen, canned, and dried fruits and fruit juices. Fruits are an important part of your healthy eating plan, and they are naturally packed with vitamins, minerals, and fiber. Fruits have a moderate amount of calories, mainly from carbohydrate, and no calories from fat. Fruits can satisfy your sweet tooth.

Fruits are excellent sources of vitamins A and C and minerals such as potassium, magnesium, folate, and copper. They are naturally low in fat and sodium and contain no cholesterol. Most fruits provide some fiber, but how much depends on the form of the fruit you eat. For example, a fresh apple provides more fiber than applesauce, and there's no fiber in apple juice.

When you vary the fruits you eat, you get the variety of vitamins and minerals they offer. Nutrition studies have shown the benefits of eating fruit (these studies usually also consider the benefits of eating more vegetables, too). Together, fruit and vegetables have been shown to reduce the risk for and help manage type 2 diabetes, high blood pressure, and heart disease. They also protect against certain cancers, such as mouth, stomach, and colon cancer.

Nutrition in Different Fruits

Different groups of fruit have different nutrition assets.

- Berries offer a good source of vitamin C and fiber.
- Citrus fruits, along with kiwi, guava, papaya, and cantaloupe, are well known for their high vitamin C content.
- Orange fruits, such as mango, apricot, red or pink grapefruit, and cantaloupe, are good sources of vitamin A.
- Oranges, bananas, dried fruits, cantaloupe, and honeydew are good sources of potassium.
- Oranges and orange juice can also tout their superior folate (folic acid) content.

Fruit: How Much People Eat

F is the grade most people get when it comes to eating fruit. The situation is even worse than it is for vegetables. Once you leave your own kitchen, it's difficult to find fruit, and if you do it's so expensive that you may resist the purchase. Fruit isn't plentiful at fast-food or sit-down restaurants. Fruit is often an afterthought after or between meals, if you even remember to eat it at all. If you aren't at home, the lack of available fruit presents challenges. People also don't vary their choices of fruits enough—it's apples, oranges, and bananas. Yet, a greater variety of fruits are available in the supermarket year round.

The excuses for not eating enough fruit are similar to the excuses for not eating enough vegetables. You may think that fruits are too much trouble, or you don't have any around when you're hungry. Interestingly, in today's fast-paced world, fruit is an ideal food. It requires no preparation—just wash and eat. Too often, however, fruit is left to rot. We find it easier to buy candy bars, potato chips, or sandwich crackers. Why? Because fruit is not for sale where and when we want it—in convenience stores, sandwich or coffee shops, or fast-food restaurants. Today, more fruit is being sold in these venues; however, it is often sold in large containers of mixed fruit or by the piece. Not to mention that it's priced so high that it's easy to say no.

You might not buy fresh fruit because it gets soft and brown before you eat it—the same problem you might have with vegetables. Then, you don't have fruit in the house when you want it. If you don't eat breakfast at home, you miss the ripe opportunity for a few slices of banana or peaches on cereal or raisins in your oatmeal. When it comes to a late-night taste of "something sweet," ice cream, frozen yogurt, or custard wins out over fruit.

Get to Know Yourself

If you want to change your eating habits, learn what you eat now. Ask yourself these questions about fruits:

- How many servings of fruit do I eat on average each day? Is this enough or too much?

- What fruits do I eat? Is it a narrow or varied list?
- What forms of fruits do I buy?
- Do I buy and drink a lot of fruit juice?
- Do I think fruit causes problems with my blood glucose levels?

How Many Servings of Fruits for You?

In chapter 6, you determined that a certain calorie range was the best for you. Find that calorie range in the chart on the next page and then spot the number of servings of fruits you need each day. It is somewhere between 3 and 5. This might seem like a lot of fruit to eat, and it is probably more than you currently eat. In this chapter, you'll learn easy ways to eat more fruit.

Get to Know Your Serving Sizes

The chart on pages 136–138 at the end of this chapter shows serving sizes for many fruits you commonly eat, along with their calories, carbohydrate, and fiber. Check the chart for exact amounts because there is variation. Each fruit serving, on average, contains about 15 grams of carbohydrates and 60 calories.

In general, 1 fruit serving =
- one small or half a large piece of fruit
- 1/2 cup canned fruit packed with no sugar added or unsweetened fruit juice
- 1/4 cup dried fruit.

It's important to eat the correct serving size, and it's easy to eat pieces of fruit that are more than one serving. Weigh and measure your foods on occasion to make sure you're estimating correctly and try to buy consistent sizes of fruit.

Find Your Calorie Range

Which category fits you?	Women who…	Women who…	Women who…	Children	Teen boys
	• want to lose weight • are small in size • and/or are sedentary	• are older and smaller • are larger and want to lose weight • and/or are sedentary	• are moderate to large size Men who… • are older • are small to moderate size and want to lose weight	Teen girls Women who… • are larger size and active Men who… • are small to moderate size and are at desired body weight	Men who… • are active and moderate to large size
Daily calorie range	1,200–1,400	1,400–1,600	1,600–1,900	1,900–2,300	2,300–2,800
How Many Servings of Fruits Do You Need Each Day?					
Fruits	3	3	3	4	5

Sample Meal Plan

The sample meal plan on page 131 gives you an idea of how to fit three servings of fruits into your day. The sample is designed for a person who needs 1,400–1,600 calories a day. Chapter 5 provides sample plans for other calorie ranges, along with nutritional information for several plans.

Best Form of Fruit to Eat

Fruit is your best bet if you're trying to eat the maximum amount of fiber. When possible, choose fresh fruit. Fruit that is canned or packaged with no sugar added or sweetened with a no-calorie sweetener, such as applesauce, is certainly a healthy alternative when fresh is not available. Dried fruits, such as raisins, apricots, dried apples, dates, and the like, are excellent sources of nutrition. They are not as perishable as fresh fruit, and they offer a good option for carry-along snacks; however, they are concentrated sources of carbohydrate, and it's easy to eat too much.

It is a good idea to drink as little fruit juice as possible. Fruit juice does offer good nutrition, especially if it is fortified with extra nutrition, such as Vitamin D and calcium, but it doesn't offer the fiber of fresh fruit. Plus, if you're quenching your thirst it can be challenging to drink only the small amount in one or two servings of fruit juice. A typical jar of juice from a convenience store is 12 or 16 ounces—that's 3 to 4 fruit servings. If you choose to drink juice, at least make sure it is fortified with additional nutrients, such as calcium and vitamin D.

Fruit and Blood Glucose

People with diabetes often have questions about eating fruit: Will fruit juice raise my blood glucose levels more quickly than a piece of fruit? Should I avoid fruit in the morning because my blood glucose

One-Day Meal Plan: 1,400–1,600 Calories

BREAKFAST

1/2 whole grain bagel (2 oz) with	2 starches
1 1/2 Tbsp light cream cheese	1 fat
3/4 cup blueberries with	**1 fruit**
1/3 cup plain fat-free yogurt	1/2 milk

LUNCH

Tuna salad made with	
2 oz tuna (1/2 cup), water-packed	2 oz meat
1 Tbsp light mayonnaise	1 fat
2 Tbsp diced celery	1 vegetable
1 Tbsp diced onions	
Tomato slices	
2 slices whole-wheat bread	2 starches
1 cup raw or blanched broccoli	1 vegetable
1 cup fat-free milk	1 milk
1/2 large apple	**1 fruit**

DINNER

3 oz grilled salmon with	3 oz meat
lemon and herbs	free food
Stir-fried vegetables with	
1/4 cup onions, cooked	2 vegetables
1/2 cup snow peas, cooked	
1/2 cup red peppers, cooked	
2 tsp canola oil	2 fats
1 cup brown rice	3 starches

EVENING SNACK

Mix together:	
1/2 cup crushed canned pineapple	**1 fruit**
(packed in own juice)	
1/3 cup plain fat-free yogurt	1/2 milk
1/8 cup chopped pecans	2 fats

might be higher then than at other times in the day? Is it better to eat fruit with meals rather than with snacks?

The effect of fruit on your blood glucose depends on many factors:
- the form of the fruit—is it juice that you gulp in seconds or a piece of fresh fruit that takes a few minutes to eat?
- whether you eat the fruit as part of a meal, at the end of the meal, or by itself as a snack
- the glycemic index (GI) or glycemic load of the fruit (see chapter 4).

In general, fruit does not raise blood glucose faster than other sources of carbohydrate; however, some fruits can raise your blood glucose faster than others if eaten alone. According to some GI rankings, apples, grapefruit, prunes, and peaches have a low GI, whereas dates, pineapple, raisins, and watermelon have a higher GI.

The challenge is to determine how fruit in general and specific fruits affect your blood glucose: Does eating fruit in the morning make it more difficult for you to keep your blood glucose on target throughout the day? Does one particular kind of fruit send your blood glucose soaring? Does a piece of fruit as an afternoon snack give you just enough carbohydrate to last until dinner?

Determine the fruit that is best for you to eat after considering your nutrition and your blood glucose goals. Figure out whether it's best to have fruit at meals or at snacks. Use glucose monitoring to answer your questions about how fruit works in your body. Eat the fruit and check your glucose level about 1 to 2 hours after you eat it.

Another important key is to eat the proper servings of fruit. Check out the serving sizes on pages 136–138. It's easy to drink a few extra ounces of fruit juice or to call a huge piece of fruit one serving when it is really two or more.

● **QUICK TIP**

The bottom line is that fruit is a source of energy, vitamins, minerals, and fiber not to be missed. Try to eat fruit each day.

Tips for Buying, Preparing, and Eating More Fruits

- Take advantage of the pre-cut, ready-to-eat fruit available in today's supermarkets. This makes it easy to have fruit at the ready.
- Add berries to cereal, plain yogurt, or light sour cream or use them to top pancakes, waffles, ice cream, or frozen yogurt. Add slices of banana or peaches to cold cereal.
- Add raisins, pieces of dried apricot, or chopped apple when cooking hot cereal.
- Keep a plastic container full of cut-up fruit, so you can have some at breakfast or for a snack topped with plain or fruited fat-free yogurt (for more calcium).
- Take one or two pieces of fruit from home each day to eat with lunch, as an afternoon snack, or on your way home to take the edge off your hunger.
- Keep dried fruit, raisins, figs, apricots, peaches, or pears around to use for a snack, for fuel on long hikes or bike rides, or to stash in your desk or locker. (Watch your serving size.)
- Keep canned or jarred fruit with no sugar added in the pantry—applesauce, peaches, pears, and pineapple for starters.
- Keep frozen fruit with no added sugar around. Blend it into a breakfast shake or smoothie or use as a topping for ice cream or frozen yogurt.
- Toss fruit into entrées—pineapple in stir-fry or on pizza, fresh or dried cranberries or peaches in chicken dishes, or apricots or apples in pork dishes.
- Serve fruit with the main course—applesauce with pork chops or roast, pineapple with ham, homemade cranberry sauce with chicken.

Dress Up Fruit for Dessert

Fruit makes a great dessert, from apple cobbler to key lime pie. The problem is that many calories and grams of fat and carbohydrate are added before the dessert enters your mouth. The chart below gives a few examples of how fruit can be a healthy low-calorie dessert or a less healthy high-calorie one.

Your challenge is to search for ways to prepare fruits to satisfy your sweet tooth but not add a notch to your belt buckle. Start with these:

- baked apples, low-calorie apple cobbler, or applesauce
- banana bread, frozen bananas rolled in cocoa or chopped nuts
- sliced bananas or canned peaches or pears in fat-free, sugar-free pudding mix
- frozen (no-sugar-added) blueberries or strawberries on frozen yogurt or topped with plain yogurt
- frozen (no-sugar-added) blueberries or strawberries on angel food cake
- sliced fresh fruit or fruit kabobs dipped in fruited yogurt or other low-calorie dip

High-Calorie and Low-Calorie Dessert Choices

Food	Serving	Calories	Fat (g)
Apple crisp	1 cup	194	8
Apple (medium), peeled and baked with low-calorie sweetener and cinnamon	1	73	0
Banana cream pie	1 piece	398	20
Banana bread	1 slice	120	5
Strawberry ice cream	1 cup	254	11
Strawberries (frozen) on 1 piece angel food cake	1/2 cup	194	0

David's Story

David is 48 years old and has had type 2 diabetes for 8 years. When he was diagnosed, he was told to eat healthy foods and to avoid too many sweets. Recently, he began to have some vision problems and was feeling the symptoms of thirst and tiredness.

David's doctor found that his blood glucose was high, and his A1C was 9.4%. This means that his blood glucose had been averaging around 220 mg/dl. His blood pressure was also high, at 195/90 mmHg. David's doctor suggested that he begin taking a blood glucose-lowering medication to lower his blood glucose and a blood pressure medication. He gave him a list of dietitians who might be able to help him slim down and cut back on sodium.

David and the dietitian discussed what he usually eats and drinks, and David was surprised to see what his food "habits" were. David is a construction worker and, in the warm climate, he gets thirsty on the job. He has been drinking fruit and sports drinks to quench his thirst. He eats one piece of fruit a day—maybe a small banana on a bowl of cereal. If he's on the run, breakfast becomes a plain donut or two and coffee in his truck on the way to the job. He might eat a piece of fruit in the evening.

David's dietitian explained that the fruit and sports drinks contain lots of sugars and calories and not much in the way of nutrition. She suggested that he quench his thirst with water, mineral water, iced tea, or diet lemonade. The RD gave David the idea of cutting up grapefruit, apples, and oranges, once a week and putting them in a container in the refrigerator. Then he would have ready access to fruit salad each morning or as a snack at night. She suggested he put a few tablespoons of fat-free, sugar-free fruited yogurt or, better yet, plain yogurt on the fruit to get in much needed dairy foods and some calcium.

To increase the number of fruit servings per day, David said he'd be willing to eat a piece of fruit before he leaves for work and keep servings of dried fruit in his glove compartment to eat one serving of it in the afternoon. He will try for a third serving of fruit as part of an evening snack of cereal and milk or yogurt and ginger snaps.

Serving Sizes for Fruits

Food	Serving Size	Calories	Carb (g)	Fiber (g)
FRESH/CANNED/DRIED FRUITS				
Apple, with peel	1 small (4 oz)	54	14.4	2.5
Apples, dried	4 rings	63	17.1	2.3
Applesauce, unsweetened	1/2 cup	52	13.8	1.5
Apricots, canned, juice pack	1/2 cup, halves	59	15.1	2.0
Apricots, dried	8 halves	67	17.5	2.0
Apricots, fresh	4 apricots	67	15.6	3.4
Banana, fresh	1 extra small (<6" long)	72	18.5	2.1
Blackberries, fresh	3/4 cup	56	13.8	5.7
Blueberries, dried	2 tbsps	69	16.0	1.0
Blueberries, fresh	3/4 cup	62	15.8	2.6
Cantaloupe melon, fresh	1 cup	56	13.4	1.3
Cherries, canned, juice pack, sweet	1/2 cup	68	17.3	1.9
Cherries, sweet, fresh	12 cherries	59	13.6	1.9
Cherries, dried	2 tbsps	66	16.0	1.0
Cranberries, dried	2 tbsps	47	12.5	0.9
Dates	3 dates	69	18.5	1.9

Figs, dried	1 1/2 figs	71	18.2	2.8
Figs, fresh	2 medium (2 1/4" dia)	74	19.2	3.3
Fruit cocktail, canned, juice pack	1/2 cup	60	14.0	1.0
Grapefruit sections, canned	3/4 cup	69	17.2	0.7
Grapefruit, fresh	1/2 grapefruit	53	13.4	1.8
Grapes, fresh seedless, small	17 grapes	60	15.1	0.8
Honeydew melon, fresh	1 cup, diced	61	15.5	1.4
Kiwi	1 fruit without skin, large	56	13.3	2.7
Mandarin oranges, canned, juice pack	3/4 cup	69	17.9	1.3
Mango, fresh	1/2 mango, small	68	17.7	1.9
Nectarine, fresh	1 small (5 oz)	60	14.3	2.3
Orange, fresh	1 orange	62	15.4	3.1
Papaya, fresh	1 cup, cubes	55	13.7	2.5
Peach, fresh	1 medium	57	14.0	1.9
Peaches, canned, juice pack	1/2 cup	55	14.3	1.6
Pear, fresh	1/2 large (approx 2 per lb)	61	16.2	3.2
Pears, canned, juice pack	1/2 cup	62	16.0	2.0
Pineapple, canned, juice pack	1/2 cup	74	19.5	1.0

(continues)

Adapted from *Choose Your Foods: Exchange Lists for Diabetes* (American Dietetic Association and American Diabetes Association, 2008).

Serving Sizes for Fruits *(continued)*

Food	Serving Size	Calories	Carb (g)	Fiber (g)
Pineapple, fresh	3/4 cup	56	14.7	1.6
Plum, fresh	2 plum (2 1/8" dia)	61	15.1	1.8
Plums, canned, juice pack	1/2 cup	73	19.1	1.3
Plums, dried (prunes)	3 prunes	60	15.6	1.8
Raisins, dark, seedless	2 tbsps	54	14.2	0.7
Raspberries, fresh	1 cup	60	14.2	8.4
Strawberries, fresh	1 1/4 cups	57	13.3	4.4
Tangerine, fresh	2 small	81	20.3	2.7
Watermelon, fresh	1 1/4 cups	57	14.3	0.8
FRUIT JUICES				
Apple juice or cider, canned or bottle	1/2 cup	58	14.5	0.1
Fruit juice blends, 100% juice	1/3 cup	50	11.6	0.1
Grape juice	1/3 cup	50	12.5	0.1
Grapefruit juice, canned	1/2 cup	47	11.1	0.1
Orange juice, fresh	1/2 cup	56	12.9	0.2
Pineapple juice, canned	1/2 cup	70	17.2	0.3
Prune juice, bottled	1/3 cup	59	14.7	0.9

Adapted from *Choose Your Foods: Exchange Lists for Diabetes* (American Dietetic Association and American Diabetes Association, 2008).

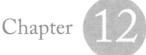
Milk and Yogurt

What You'll Learn:

- the foods in the milk and yogurt group and their nutrition assets
- healthy eating goals for the milk and yogurt food group
- a frame of reference for how much dairy foods people eat
- questions to ask yourself to get to know your current habits
- the number of servings of milk or yogurt to eat based on your calorie needs
- the dairy, calcium, and osteoporosis connection
- tips to help you buy, prepare, and eat more milk and yogurt
- the serving sizes and nutrition numbers for milk and yogurt

Foods in the Milk and Yogurt Group

This group includes mainly milk and yogurt. Dairy products that contain little to no calcium, such as cream cheese, cream, and butter, are generally found in the fat group. You'll find cheese in the meat and meat substitute group because, other than being a great source of calcium, cheese has more in common nutritionally with meats containing mainly protein and fat.

Milk and yogurt that are fat-free are a nice combination package of carbohydrate and protein. You may not often think of milk and yogurt as sources of carbohydrate, but an 8-ounce glass of milk contains almost as much carbohydrate as a slice of bread or 1/2 cup of pasta. Milk and yogurt also pack in about as much protein as one ounce of meat. If you use fat-free products, they come with nearly no saturated fat, trans fat, or cholesterol. Milk and yogurt do poorly in the fiber department but are excellent sources of many vitamins and minerals.

They beat all other food groups for calcium. In addition, they're good sources of riboflavin, magnesium, phosphorus, and potassium. Because most milk today is fortified with vitamins A and D, it's an important source of these fat-soluble vitamins, as well. If you eat the needed three servings a day from the milk and yogurt group, you're much more likely to get an adequate amount of these nutrients.

Host of Health Benefits

Healthy bones and the prevention of osteoporosis are well-known benefits of sufficient calcium. Over the last few years, even more health benefits have been attributed to dairy foods. Sufficient intake of dairy foods has been linked to better control of blood pressure as well as to weight control.

Osteoporosis

More than 40 million people in America have osteoporosis, and more are estimated to have low bone mass (osteopenia), which places them at increased risk for osteoporosis. Osteopenia and osteoporosis are more common in women and older adults. Osteoporosis is a breaking down of the bones that leaves bones thinner and more brittle and puts people at increased risk of bone fractures. Hip fractures are the most common fracture people incur. Anyone can get osteoporosis; however, smaller women who have less bone mass are at greater risk.

Tips to Prevent Osteoporosis

The best way to prevent osteoporosis is to get enough calcium throughout your life, so speak to your children and grandchildren about the importance of milk and yogurt.

- Get enough calcium from dairy foods and other high-calcium foods, as well as a calcium supplement with extra vitamin D to maximize calcium absorption, if necessary.
- Do weight-bearing activities—walk, jog, dance, garden, or lift light weights—a few times a week. Weight-bearing exercise helps you maintain your bone and muscle mass, especially as you age.

Blood Pressure

Several studies have shown that getting enough low-fat dairy foods can help lower blood pressure. The frequently cited DASH (Dietary Approaches to Stop Hypertension; see page 82) study reported the effects of three different eating plans on blood pressure. People who ate healthy amounts of grains, low-fat, high-calcium dairy foods (3 servings/day), fruits (4–6 servings/day), and vegetables (3–6 servings/day) lowered their blood pressure the most. Amazingly, the effect of the healthy eating plan was evident within one week and had the greatest effect on lowering blood pressure in just two weeks! For some people, the healthy eating plan reduced their blood pressure as much as one blood pressure medicine would.

Milk and Yogurt: How Americans Eat

According to the National Dairy Council (www.nationaldairycouncil. org), 75% of Americans get less than the recommended intake of three 8-ounce glasses of milk or the equivalent dairy food a day. What is of particular concern today is the low intake of dairy foods among children and teens. They are paying for this deficiency even in their younger years with a reported increase in the incidence of bone fractures. Because dairy foods are the main contributor of calcium to the diet, this insufficient intake means that many people don't get enough calcium and may suffer both immediate and long-term consequences.

Get to Know Yourself

If you want to change your eating habits, learn what you eat now. Ask yourself these questions about foods in the milk and yogurt group:

- How many servings of milk or yogurt do I eat on average each day? Is this enough or too much?
- Do I correctly estimate the servings of milk or yogurt I eat?
- What type of milk and yogurt do I buy (fat-free, 2%, or full-fat)?
- Do I get the right amount of calcium each day to meet my nutritional needs?
- Am I at risk for osteoporosis?
- Do I buy calcium-fortified foods when possible or add milk or yogurt in food preparation to get more calcium?

How Many Servings of Milk and Yogurt for You?

In chapter 6, you determined that a certain calorie range was the best for you. Find that calorie range in the chart on page 144 and then spot the number of servings of milk and yogurt you need each day. It's 2 servings a day across the board; however, you'll find in this chapter that if you can sneak in a third serving of milk or yogurt without going overboard on calories, you'll have an easier time meeting your calcium goals. If you are like most Americans, you get about 1 1/2 servings of dairy foods a day. In this chapter, you'll learn easy ways to consume more milk and yogurt.

Get to Know Your Serving Sizes

The chart on pages 152–153 at the end of the chapter shows serving sizes for milk and yogurt products in this food group, along with their calories, carbohydrate, protein, and fat content. Each serving of milk or yogurt contains about 12 grams of carbohydrates and 8 grams of protein. The amount of calories that each serving contains depends on the amount of fat. Fat-free products contain about 80 to 100 calories, whereas higher-fat products, like whole milk, contain 8 grams of fat per serving and 150 calories.

In general, 1 serving =
- 1 cup (8 oz) of any type of milk
- 2/3 to 3/4 cup of various types of yogurt.

It's important to drink and eat the right amounts of food, so you may want to measure the amount of milk and yogurt you eat occasionally to make sure you're estimating correctly. Another helpful portion-control tip is to drink and eat these foods out of the same cup or bowl as often as possible.

Sample Meal Plan

The sample meal plan on page 145 gives you an idea of how to fit two servings of milk and yogurt into your day. The sample is designed for a person who needs 1,400–1,600 calories a day. Chapter 6 provides sample plans for other calorie ranges, along with nutritional information for several plans.

Find Your Calorie Range

Which category fits you?	Women who... • want to lose weight • are small in size • and/or are sedentary	Women who... • are older and smaller • are larger and want to lose weight • and/or are sedentary	Women who... • are moderate to large size Men who... • are older • are small to moderate size and want to lose weight	Children Teen girls Women who... • are larger size and active Men who... • are small to moderate size and are at desired body weight	Teen boys Men who... • are active and moderate to large size
Daily calorie range	1,200–1,400	1,400–1,600	1,600–1,900	1,900–2,300	2,300–2,800

How Many Servings of Milk and Yogurt Do You Need Each Day?

Milk and Yogurt	2	2	2	2	2

One-Day Meal Plan: 1,400–1,600 Calories

BREAKFAST

1/2 whole grain bagel (2 oz) with	2 starches
1 1/2 Tbsp light cream cheese	1 fat
3/4 cup blueberries with	1 fruit
1/3 cup plain fat-free yogurt	**1/2 milk**

LUNCH

Tuna salad made with	
2 oz tuna (1/2 cup), water-packed	2 oz meat
1 Tbsp light mayonnaise	1 fat
2 Tbsp diced celery	1 vegetable
1 Tbsp diced onions	
Tomato slices	
2 slices whole-wheat bread	2 starches
1 cup raw or blanched broccoli	1 vegetable
1 cup fat-free milk	**1 milk**
1/2 large apple	1 fruit

DINNER

3 oz grilled salmon with	3 oz meat
lemon and herbs	free food
Stir-fried vegetables with	
1/4 cup onions, cooked	2 vegetables
1/2 cup snow peas, cooked	
1/2 cup red peppers, cooked	
2 tsp canola oil	2 fats
1 cup brown rice	3 starches

EVENING SNACK

Mix together:	
1/2 cup crushed canned pineapple	1 fruit
(packed in own juice)	
1/3 cup plain fat-free yogurt	**1/2 milk**
1/8 cup chopped pecans	2 fats

Calcium: How Much and from Which Foods?

The table below shows the current recommendations for calcium for the general public across all age ranges. People with diabetes can follow these same recommendations. The best food sources of calcium are dairy products—milk, yogurt, and cheese. Other nondairy sources of calcium are dark green leafy vegetables, such as broccoli, kale, and collards; calcium-fortified soy milk; sardines; and canned salmon.

Today, you can buy more products that are calcium-fortified. Examples of these are fruit juices, such as orange, grapefruit, and apple juice, as well as hot and cold cereals. (Chapter 6 provides a list of top ten sources of calcium per food serving.) Note that the sample meal plan above contains nearly 900 milligrams of calcium—still under the goal for most adults, but much higher than many people achieve daily.

In this meal plan, you'd reach 1,000 milligrams easily if you substituted canned salmon for tuna fish at lunch, mixed a handful of spinach or other dark green leafy vegetables into your stir-fried vegetables at dinner, used calcium-fortified fat-free milk, or took a multivitamin with at least 200 mg of calcium (usual amount).

Daily Calcium Recommendations

Age Ranges	Calcium Recommendation (mg)
Girls and boys: ages 1–3	500
Girls and boys: ages 4–8	800
Girls and boys: ages 9–18	1,300
Women and men: ages 19–50	1,000
Women: age 51 and older	1,200
Women: pregnant or breastfeeding, over age 18	1,000
Men: age 51 and older	1,000

A Maze of Milks and Yogurts

There's a maze of milks on the supermarket shelf today, from fat-free to whole milk, soy milk, lactose-free, and beyond. The best advice is to choose a variety of fat-free milk. A fat-free milk provides all the nutrition benefits with nearly no saturated and trans fats and cholesterol.

Some people think that they are taking a big leap when they move from whole milk to 2% milk, but that's not so. Whole milk has only 3 1/2% fat and about 150 calories per 8 ounces, whereas 2% has about 120 calories. Not a big difference. Fat-free milk has about 90 calories per 8 ounces. If you drink soy milk, choose a fat-free calcium-fortified type; however, you still won't get some of the other nutrition that dairy offers.

> ● QUICK TIP
>
> Take advantage of the calcium-fortified varieties of fat-free milk that are available nearly everywhere. You get 500 milligrams of calcium per 8 ounces versus 300 milligrams in regular fat-free milk. If you can't tolerate fat-free, then choose 1% milk.

If you are lactose intolerant, drink lactose-free milk. Today, you can buy calcium-fortified lactose-free milk, or you can buy a product called Lactaid that you add to milk and other lactose-containing foods. Lactaid breaks down lactose so that you may be able to eat dairy foods without problems. Try to eat vegetables and fruits that contain calcium as well. People with lactose intolerance who avoid dairy products need to take a calcium supplement. Talk to your health care provider about the best one for you.

There's also a maze of yogurts on the market today, from full-fat to non-fat or fat-free. The same advice applies for yogurt: choose the lowest-fat types. Another consideration when you buy yogurt is how it is sweetened. You can find plain yogurt that contains no added sweeteners and fruit-flavored yogurt sweetened with a no-calorie sweetener or with regular sweeteners. Once fruit is added to yogurt, the calories and carbohydrate go up. The calories go up less if the yogurt is sweetened with a no-calorie sweetener. This is true for yogurt in containers as well as yogurt drinks. Skip the sprinkles, granola, and other calorie-raising and/or nutritionally lacking additions.

Calcium on the Nutrition Facts Label

According to the Food and Drug Administration's regulations, food labels must provide daily values for two important nutrients, calcium and iron. As a result, the calcium content of many foods you buy is easy to figure because the daily value for calcium is 1,000 milligrams per day. For example, if a product contains 35% of the daily value of calcium per serving, you know that the serving provides 350 milligrams of calcium. (Learn more about daily values in chapter 7, page 65.)

People who have difficulty getting enough calcium may need to take a calcium supplement. This is especially true for women of child-bearing years, post-menopausal women, and people who eat less than 1,500 calories a day. If you do not eat enough calcium and know that, even if you try hard, you won't get enough, discuss a supplement with your health care provider. Choose a capsule, tablet, or bite-size chewable calcium supplement that provides 500 milligrams. For more information on calcium supplements, see chapter 7).

To properly use the calcium you get, it's important that you also get enough vitamin D. Vitamin D is necessary for the body to absorb calcium. If you drink sufficient milk (3 servings a day) and take a daily multivitamin and mineral supplement with 400 IU of vitamin D, you'll get enough vitamin D. However, the 400 IU recommendation might soon move upwards (see Vitamin D discussion in chapter 7). Another way to easily get more vitamin D is to buy a calcium supplement that also contains vitamin D. Many of them do.

Tips for Buying, Preparing, and Eating More Milk and Yogurt

- Opt for 8 ounces of fat-free fortified milk at meals.
- Gradually switch to fat-free milk to lower your saturated and trans fats and calories.
- Add a bit more milk to coffee or tea if you use it.
- Choose fat-free milk when you order a fancy coffee or tea drink.
- Eat more hot cereal, substitute milk for at least half (if not all) the water you use to cook the cereal, or use more milk on the cereal as you eat it.
- Eat more high-fiber dry cereals. You'll drink more milk and get a good boost of fiber. Choose cereals that are calcium-fortified.
- Don't limit cereal and milk to breakfast; it can be a quick and easy lunch, dinner, or snack. It is a great way to work in another fruit serving, too.
- Blend a milk or yogurt shake for a quick and tasty breakfast or snack. Put a serving of milk or yogurt in a blender, add a serving of fruit (banana, strawberries, or peaches), add a bit of extract (vanilla, rum, or maple), blend it up, and sip it down. If you want a cold shake, freeze the fruit before blending.
- Create your own yogurt combo. Take plain fat-free yogurt and toss in Grape-Nuts, a low-fat granola cereal, dried fruit (diced dried apricots, apples, or pears), or a few chopped nuts for a good crunch.
- Drop a few tablespoons of yogurt on fresh or canned fruit.
- Use plain yogurt as a substitute for sour cream on potatoes. Mix in fresh herbs, garlic, Dijon mustard, cayenne, or curry (or any combination of herbs and spices) for some extra kick.
- Make yogurt cheese the thickness of cream cheese and add some no-sugar jelly to spread on bagels or toast. (Do this by draining plain yogurt through cheese cloth for a few hours to drain out some of the liquid.)
- Add nonfat dry milk to recipes where the taste will blend in— meat loaf or meatballs, soups, casseroles, or gravies.
- Add fat-free milk or nonfat dry milk to eggs for scrambled eggs, omelets, or French toast.

Dorothy's Story

Dorothy, who is 33 years old and 28 weeks pregnant with her second child, just found out she has gestational diabetes (diabetes that occurs only during pregnancy). Dorothy's first child weighed 9.3 pounds at birth, and her doctor suspects she had gestational diabetes toward the end of that pregnancy. Dorothy has gained about 20 pounds since the beginning of her first pregnancy, and that is one reason her blood glucose is higher at an earlier stage of pregnancy.

Dorothy and her doctors want to keep her blood glucose on target with a healthy eating plan as long as possible; however, it is likely she will need insulin toward the end of her pregnancy. When Dorothy met with the dietitian after her diagnosis, they talked about what she eats, particularly how much milk and yogurt because of her calcium needs during pregnancy.

Dorothy sometimes has a bowl of dry cereal with 2% milk, maybe a green leafy vegetable a few times a week, and a cup of low-fat frozen yogurt about four nights a week. Dorothy gets some additional calcium from a prenatal multivitamin and mineral tablet. The RD and Dorothy saw that she is not getting the 1,000 milligrams of calcium that she needs during pregnancy; she eats about half the amount of calcium she needs.

Dorothy and her RD developed some ways that she could eat more calcium. Instead of skipping breakfast, she could make a yogurt- or milk-based breakfast shake with a banana or some berries. The RD encouraged Dorothy to eat breakfast before she leaves for work. Dry or cooked cereal with fat-free milk is a great choice, especially if she chooses calcium-fortified cereal. She should make cooked cereal with fat-free milk, not water, and then use more milk on the cooked cereal. Another quick breakfast that offers calcium is cheese toast (melted cheese on bread).

For snacks, the dietitian suggested crackers and cheese (low-fat or reduced-calorie), a nonfat fruited yogurt, plain yogurt with fresh fruit, a serving of a low-sugar and low-fat custard, or pudding. The RD gave her quick and easy recipes for custard and pudding and encouraged her to make a batch for the week. She noted that it would be enjoyed by Dorothy's whole family. These changes alone will not get Dorothy's calcium up to the level she needs. The dietitian suggested that she talk to her doctor about this and find out about taking a calcium supplement.

Finally, the RD encouraged Dorothy to schedule several follow-up visits during her pregnancy and to return after her baby is born. If Dorothy is going to breastfeed, she will also need 1,000 milligrams of calcium per day. The dietitian encouraged her to begin to slowly lose some weight after delivery, noting that nearly half of women who have gestational diabetes develop type 2 diabetes later in life. Research shows Dorothy can reduce her chances of developing pre-diabetes or type 2 diabetes if she controls her weight and walks or exercises regularly. Because she is at risk for diabetes due to her history of gestational diabetes, Dorothy needs to have her A1C checked once a year according to the ADA recommendations.

Serving Sizes for Milk and Yogurt

Food	Serving Size	Calories	Carb (g)	Fat (g)	Protein (g)
FAT-FREE MILKS/LOW-FAT MILKS					
Acidophilus milk, fat-free	1 cup	90	13.0	0.2	9.0
Buttermilk, fat-free	1 cup	98	11.7	0.0	8.1
Buttermilk, low-fat (1%)	1 cup	98	11.7	2.2	8.1
Lactaid, fat free	1 cup	80	13	0.0	8.1
Milk, 1% (low-fat)	1 cup	110	13.0	2.5	8.0
Milk, evaporated fat-free	1/2 cup	100	14.5	0.3	9.7
Milk, fat-free (nonfat, skim)	1 cup	90	13.0	0.2	9.0
Yogurt, flavored, fat-free, sweetened with Splenda	1 container (6 oz)	80	11.0	0.3	7.0
Yogurt, nonfat plain	1 container (6 oz)	82	12.0	0.3	8.2
Yogurt, plain low-fat	1 container (6 oz)	107	12.0	2.6	8.9
REDUCED-FAT MILKS					
Acidophilus milk, 2%	1 cup	128	11.2	4.7	7.9
Kefir, made with 2% milk	1 cup	120	13.0	4.6	9.0
Lactaid, reduced-fat	1 cup	130	13.0	5.0	7.9
Milk, reduced-fat (2%)	1 cup	130	12.0	5.0	8.1

WHOLE MILKS					
Milk, evaporated whole	1/2 cup	169	12.7	9.5	8.6
Milk, goat, whole	1 cup	168	10.9	10.1	8.7
Milk, whole	1 cup	150	12.0	8.0	8.0
Yogurt, plain, made from whole milk	1 cup	160	12.0	8.0	9.0
DAIRY-LIKE FOODS					
Chocolate milk, fat-free	1 cup	160	31.0	0.0	9.0
Chocolate milk, whole	1 cup	208	25.9	8.5	7.9
Eggnog, whole milk	1/2 cup	171	17.2	9.5	4.8
Rice drink, fat-free or 1%, plain	1 cup	90	18.0	1.5	1.1
Rice drink, low-fat, flavored	1 cup	122	25.0	2.0	1.0
Smoothie, regular, yogurt-based, flavored	1 container (10 fl oz)	260	49.7	3.3	8.0
Soy milk, light	1 cup (8 fl oz)	100	15.0	2.0	5.0
Soy milk, regular, plain	1 cup	115	11.0	4.1	8.0
Yogurt and juice blend	1 cup	150	34.0	0.0	3.0
Yogurt, low-carb, sweetened with Splenda	1 container (6 oz)	70	5.0	3.0	5.0
Yogurt with fruit, low-fat	1 container (6 oz)	150	28.0	1.5	6.0

Adapted from *Choose Your Foods: Exchange Lists for Diabetes* (American Dietetic Association and American Diabetes Association, 2008).

Chapter 13

Meat and Meat Substitutes

What You'll Learn:

- the foods in the meat and meat substitutes food group
- the nutrition assets and liabilities of meat and meat substitutes
- healthy eating goals for the meat and meat substitutes group
- a frame of reference for how much meat and meat substitutes people eat
- questions to ask yourself to get to know your current habits
- the number of ounces of meat to eat based on your calorie needs
- tips to help you buy, prepare, and eat healthier sources and smaller amounts of meat and meat substitutes
- the serving sizes and nutrition numbers for meat and meat substitutes

Foods in the Meat and Meat Substitutes Group

This group, often loosely referred to as the "meat" group, contains the foods that provide you with most of the protein you eat, especially if you are a vegetarian (see chapter 4). Here are the foods in the meat group: meats (red meats—beef, lamb, veal, pork); poultry (chicken, turkey); seafood (shellfish and fish); eggs; cheese; nut spreads, such as peanut and cashew butter (note: nuts are in the fat group); plant-based protein foods (legumes such as lentils, refried beans, also found in the starch group); and soy-based foods (burgers, tempeh, and tofu).

Nutrition Assets and Liabilities

This is the first food group for which a key nutrition message is to eat less. It's also the first time nutrition liabilities as well as assets are noted. The calories from foods in the meat group come from protein and varying amounts of fat. Very lean meats provide calories mainly from protein, whereas high-fat meats provide a similar amount of protein but much more fat.

The nutrition liabilities of the higher-fat meats are their fat content, as well as their saturated fat, trans fat, and cholesterol content. Both saturated and trans fat and cholesterol can raise your LDL (bad cholesterol) and blood lipid levels.

● **QUICK TIP**

According to ADA recommendations, saturated fat should represent no more than 7% of your calories, and trans fats should be as close to zero as possible.

Full-fat cheese (regular, not reduced or low fat) and beef contribute the most saturated fat to the average person's diet. Poultry contributes some, but it's way down on the list. Choosing lean beef and low-fat cheese can make a big dent in your saturated fat intake. Animal products, many of which are in this food group, contribute about 20% of trans fat. Eating less of these foods will lower the amount of trans fat you eat. Eighty percent of trans fat is from fats and commercially prepared foods with partially hydrogenated oils. Learn more about trans fats in chapter 14, page 192.

Cholesterol is only found in foods of animal origin, so it stands to reason that many foods in the meat group contain cholesterol. Foods with the highest cholesterol counts are whole eggs (it's the yolk that contains the cholesterol), organ meats, calamari (squid), and shrimp. All meats, cheese, poultry, and seafood contain some cholesterol. Foods that are high in saturated fat aren't necessarily high in cholesterol. Learn more in chapter 14.

Meats have plenty of nutrition assets. Your body needs protein, and meat provides the amino acids—the building blocks of protein—to maintain your bones, muscles, enzymes, and hormones. Red meats, like beef, veal, lamb, and pork, as well as seafood and poultry, provide good sources of several vitamins and minerals, such as iron, zinc, thiamin, riboflavin, niacin, magnesium, phosphorus, and vitamins E, B-6, and B-12. Cheese is an excellent source of calcium. Fatty fish, such as salmon, tuna, and mackerel, are good sources of the healthy omega-3 fats. Foods in the meat group have been shown to take longer to digest and, therefore, keep you feeling fuller or satiated longer.

Meats: How People Eat

People generally eat too much protein—about double what's necessary for good health. Historically, dining on large servings of meat has been a way to show wealth. Meats tend to be the focal point of meals—a three-egg omelet with cheese and sausage for breakfast, a mile-high deli sandwich packed with six or more ounces of meat for lunch, and eight or more ounces of rib eye steak for dinner. The health advice of many nutrition experts today is to consume smaller amounts of meats and make them lean.

A way to eat smaller portions is to follow the lead of other cultures. Consider Chinese stir-fry, in which small tidbits of meat are scattered among a greater amount of vegetables and served with rice, or Mexican chili, in which a tomato and bean base has bits of meat or sausage in it. Along with eating too much meat, people tend to choose meats that are higher in total fat and saturated fat than is healthy, such as full-fat cheese, marbled red meat, and sausage or bacon.

Get to Know Yourself

If you want to change your eating habits, learn what you eat now. Ask yourself these questions about meats:

- How many times a day do I eat meat?
- Do I believe I need to eat a food from the meat group at every meal?
- What cuts of meat do I buy? Are they high in fat or lean?
- Do I pull the skin off of poultry?
- Do I consume enough fish, particularly fish high in omega-3 fats, each week?
- What cooking methods and sauces and seasonings do I use to prepare meats?
- What is my typical portion of meats at breakfast, lunch, dinner, and snack time at home and at restaurants? (Weigh a few of your portions to make sure.)

How Many Servings of Meats?

In chapter 5, you saw that a certain calorie range was the best for you. Find that calorie range in the chart on page 160, and then spot the number of ounces of meat you need each day. It is somewhere between 4 and 8 ounces. Yes, you could easily eat this amount in one sitting, but this is enough meat for an entire day.

Get to Know Your Serving Sizes

The chart on pages 170–179 at the end of the chapter shows the calories, protein, total fat, saturated fat, and cholesterol per ounce in the meat and meat substitutes you commonly eat. An ounce of meat has about 7 grams of protein, no matter what kind of meat it is.

In general, a serving of meat = 2 to 3 ounces cooked.

You can see how the sources of meats you choose, day in and day out, greatly affect the calories and the amount of fat you eat. It's important to eat the correct servings of meats, so you may want to weigh and measure your foods on occasion to make sure you're estimating correctly.

Sample Meal Plan

The sample meal plan on page 162 gives you an idea of how to fit 5 ounces of meats into your day. The sample plan is designed for a person who needs 1,400–1,600 calories a day. Chapter 6 provides sample plans for other calorie ranges, along with nutritional information for several plans.

Meat and Diabetes

Learn more about how much protein and fat you need in chapter 4. The biggest reason to eat smaller portions of meat and to change the types of meat you select is to cut down on total fat, saturated fat, trans fat, and cholesterol. As a person with diabetes, you are at risk for, or may already have, heart disease and high blood pressure. A reduction in saturated fat intake and cholesterol can help you improve your blood lipid levels.

Find Your Calorie Range

Which category fits you?	Women who... • want to lose weight • are small in size and/or are sedentary	Women who... • are older and smaller • are larger and want to lose weight • and/or are sedentary	Women who... • are moderate to large size Men who... • are older • are small to moderate size and want to lose weight	Children Teen girls Women who... • are larger size and active Men who... • are small to moderate size and are at desired body weight	Teen boys Men who... • are active and moderate to large size
Daily calorie range	1,200–1,400	1,400–1,600	1,600–1,900	1,900–2,300	2,300–2,800
How Many Servings of Meats or Meat Substitutes Do You Need Each Day?					
Meat and meat substitutes	4 oz	5 oz	6 oz	7 oz	8 oz

Fat and Calories in Meat Group

What makes the calorie difference in the various types of meats and meat substitutes is the amount of fat they contain. Think of them fitting into four subgroups.

Type of Meat	Fat (g)*	Calories*	Examples
Lean	0–3	45	Poultry (without skin), beef (tenderloin, sirloin, or ground round), or seafood (salmon, tuna, tilapia, or shellfish)
Medium-fat	4–7	75	Ground beef (not lean 80/20), prime beef, pork cutlet, egg, cheese (string, feta, part-skim, reduced-fat)
High-fat	8+	100	Pork spare ribs, bacon, and regular cheese
Plant-based	Varies+	Varies+	Legumes

*Nutrition information is per 1 ounce cooked or as eaten portion.

+Plant-based protein often contains some carbohydrate. The amount of fat and calories varies.

Adapted from Choose Your Foods: Exchange Lists for Diabetes, ADA, 2008.

Choosing Healthy Meats

Beyond eating too much meat, people choose too many meats from animal sources and not enough from plant-based sources. Consider the animal sources, such as beef, eggs, cheese, seafood, and poultry, versus the plant-based sources, such as legumes and nuts. A higher consumption of animal sources leads to higher than desirable amounts of saturated and trans fats and cholesterol. This is not true for plant-based sources.

Choose lean sources of meats, prepare them in low-fat ways, and eat them in smaller amounts. Also, begin to consider making meat a side dish rather than your main entrée. Think about meat taking up no more than one quarter of your plate. This way, you'll have more room for healthy starches, fruits, and vegetables.

One-Day Meal Plan: 1,400–1,600 Calories

BREAKFAST

1/2 whole grain bagel (2 oz) with	2 starches
1 1/2 Tbsp light cream cheese	1 fat
3/4 cup blueberries with	1 fruit
1/3 cup plain fat-free yogurt	1/2 milk

LUNCH

Tuna salad made with	
2 oz tuna (1/2 cup), water-packed	**2 oz meat**
1 Tbsp light mayonnaise	1 fat
2 Tbsp diced celery	1 vegetable
1 Tbsp diced onions	
Tomato slices	
2 slices whole-wheat bread	2 starches
1 cup raw or blanched broccoli	1 vegetable
1 cup fat-free milk	1 milk
1/2 large apple	1 fruit

DINNER

3 oz grilled salmon with	**3 oz meat**
lemon and herbs	free food
Stir-fried vegetables with	
1/4 cup onions, cooked	2 vegetables
1/2 cup snow peas, cooked	
1/2 cup red peppers, cooked	
2 tsp canola oil	2 fats
1 cup brown rice	3 starches

EVENING SNACK

Mix together:	
1/2 cup crushed canned pineapple (packed in own juice)	1 fruit
1/3 cup plain fat-free yogurt	1/2 milk
1/8 cup chopped pecans	2 fats

Choose Lean

Some meats you purchase raw and cook, such as red meats, poultry, and fish. Others, such as canned tuna, cheese, and luncheon meats, you purchase ready-to-eat.

Red Meat. Choose lean options for all types of meat. Select-grade meats are leanest, choice cuts contain moderate fat, and prime cuts contain the most fat. Regardless of grade, look for well-trimmed cuts or trim them well before you cook them.

Type of Red Meat	Leaner Cuts	Higher-Fat Cuts
Beef	Round steaks and roasts (round eye, top round, bottom round, round tip), top loin, top sirloin, chuck shoulder and arm roasts, flank steak, skirt steak, top loin, ground beef (90% lean meat or greater)	Rib eye steak, rib roast, short ribs, ground beef (less than 90% lean)
Lamb	Leg, loin chop	Ground lamb, blade
Pork	Loin, tenderloin, center loin, butterfly-cut chops, loin rib chops, ham	Spare ribs, country ribs, sausage, bacon
Veal	Cutlet, rib, or loin chop	Breast

Poultry. Chicken and turkey are lower in fat than most red meats and contain less saturated fat, particularly when you remove the skin. Purchase chicken or turkey without skin or remove the skin before you cook it. White-meat chicken (the breast) is lower in fat than dark-meat (thigh and leg) by a small margin; however, if you enjoy dark meat more, the difference isn't that great. If you purchase cooked chicken and turkey, remove the skin and as much fat as possible before you eat it. More turkey products are available today, including turkey cutlets and breast, ground turkey, and turkey sausage. These are most often lower in fat than their red meat cousins. When possible, use them to replace red meat or to replace some of the red meat. For example, if you make a meatloaf, consider using half lean ground beef and half ground turkey. Duck and cornish hen are higher in fat than chicken and turkey.

Seafood. Most shellfish and fish are lower in fat and saturated fat than red meat; however, their fat content can vary. Some of the white fishes—flounder, sole, haddock—are very lean, whereas salmon, mackerel, and bluefish have more fat. Some of the fat in these fattier fish is the healthier omega-3 fat. Buy tuna packed in water rather than tuna packed in oil, and enjoy canned salmon as a healthy alternative to tuna.

Luncheon and Breakfast Meats. At the deli counter and when you order a sandwich, choose lean. Opt for turkey or smoked turkey, turkey ham, roast beef, or ham. Avoid high-fat luncheon meats like salami, bologna, and capacola. Also avoid mixed-up salads like tuna fish, seafood, and egg salad. These tend to be loaded with mayonnaise. Choose lean hotdogs or those made from turkey. When you eat breakfast meat, such as sausage or bacon, try to find lean and low-fat options. Look for turkey bacon or sausage. Many luncheon meats, hotdogs, and breakfast meats are high in sodium.

Cheese. Full-fat cheese tops the list when it comes to saturated fat. If you are a big cheese eater—say, a couple of ounces a day—save calories and grams of fat and saturated fat with healthier choices. Today, more cheeses are available in reduced-fat, part-skim, low-fat, and fat-free versions. When you buy cheese, choose a lower-fat version as long as you enjoy the taste. It's easy to find lower-fat versions of many hard and soft cheeses, such as mozzarella, Jarlsberg, ricotta, and cottage cheese. You may be able to get away with some of the hard and soft fat-free versions to combine in foods when you cook, but their taste may be lacking when it comes to just eating a piece of cheese.

Prepare Low Fat

Whether the healthier meat you have chosen is still low fat when it gets to the table depends on how you prepare it. Do you trim the fat off red meat and cook it in a way that lets the fat drip off? Do you take tuna packed in water and load it with mayonnaise or just flake it onto an entrée salad for a portion of meat? Do you barbecue chicken or deep-fry it? Do you bake a piece of flounder with lemon and herbs or bread it and fry it?

To keep your meats low in calories, learn to use low-fat preparation techniques. In other words, don't add a lot of oil, butter, mayonnaise, or cream in preparation. Learn to use low- or no-calorie sauces, flavorings, and seasonings. Use a cooking method that drips and drains fat rather than adds it, such as barbecuing, grilling, or poaching.

Tips to Reduce Fat Through Preparation

- Grill with different flavored wood chips—for example, mesquite or hickory.
- Poach in broth, garlic, herbs, wine, sherry, or any combination of flavors.
- Marinate meat, chicken, or fish for at least several hours in fat-free ingredients before cooking. For starters, try sherry, mustard, and garlic; soy or teriyaki sauce (sodium is high); ginger and garlic; vinegar (any variety); or garlic and basil.
- Make low-fat gravy using the drippings from baking or roasting as follows: Refrigerate the drippings until the fat turns solid and floats on top. Remove the fat. Then put drippings in a pan, add a bit of flour or cornstarch with a whisk, and heat to thicken. Puree any celery, onion, or carrots that were in the roasting pan and add to defatted gravy mixture to thicken. You may want to purchase a gravy defatter that allows you to pour the juices out and leave the fat in the container.
- Use salsa or pico de gallo to spice up ground beef, chicken, or shrimp for fajitas, burritos, or soft tacos.
- Mix plain fat-free yogurt with mustard and dill to top fish.
- Make low-fat tartar sauce with low-fat or fat-free mayonnaise and relish.

Eat Less

Downsize Your Portions. If your usual portion of meat, whether ham in a sandwich or several lamb chops, has typically been more than 6, 8, or 10 ounces, then 3 ounces will seem tiny. To have long-term success, you need to downsize slowly, 1 ounce at a time. If you usually eat 5 or 6 ounces of turkey in a sandwich, step down to 4 ounces and then to 3 ounces, month by month. Stuff sandwiches with lettuce, tomato, sliced cucumber, and sprouts. When you downsize servings, weigh items more frequently to help your eye adjust. Even if your servings are a bit larger than desirable in the beginning, choosing lean cuts and preparing food in low-fat ways are moves in a healthy direction.

Weigh and Measure. It is important to weigh protein foods. Use a food scale at least occasionally to make sure your portions are just right and don't keep inching up. It is easy to cut a slightly bigger wedge of cheese or eat an extra ounce of meat in a sandwich. The more often you weigh your portions of meat before they go in your mouth, the more often you'll eat the correct portion. Plus, you'll be better able to guess portions at restaurants.

Another way to estimate portions of meat is to think in terms of common objects. The palm of your hand—both width and depth—is about the size of a 3-ounce piece of meat. You can also think of a standard deck of playing cards or computer mouse to figure 3 ounces of cooked meat.

Another portion control tip is to think about the portions you want to eat when you purchase foods in the supermarket. For example, if you buy lean turkey for sandwiches and you want to make 4 sandwiches, each with 3 ounces of turkey, then buy 12 ounces. If you buy too much, then you are likely to overeat. Apply this same logic to all the meats, poultry, and seafood you buy and control your portions before you even put the food on the table. Learn more techniques for controlling the portions of meats in chapter 21.

Measuring from Raw to Cooked

Here are quick rules of thumb to translate from raw to cooked servings:

- Raw meat with no bone: 4 ounces raw = 3 ounces cooked
- Raw meat with bone: 5 ounces raw = 3 ounces cooked
- Raw poultry with skin: skin is 1/4–1/2 ounce per 4–5 ounces raw. (Remove skin before cooking or before serving to reduce the fat, saturated fat, and cholesterol content.)

When you order meats in restaurants, observe that they refer to the raw weight. For example a quarter-pound hamburger equals 3 ounces cooked; a 10-ounce T-bone steak equals about 6 ounces cooked.

Easy Ways to Eat Less

Tips to choose smaller portions:

- Split sandwiches in restaurants. Ask for two extra pieces of bread or an extra roll and split the meat from one sandwich into two.
- Split a meat entrée in restaurants. The usual portion you are served in sit-down restaurants is 6 to 8 or more ounces. This is plenty for two. If you need more food, fill the meal out with an extra salad, cooked vegetable, or healthy starch.
- Make room on your plate for starches and vegetables, so that the smaller-than-usual piece of meat won't seem so small.
- Buy and prepare smaller quantities (just what you need for the recipe) so that you eat less.
- Cook dishes that stretch the meat portion—Chinese stir-fry, pasta with meat sauce, or beef and bean burritos.
- Load sandwiches with raw vegetables. (It's easier with pita bread because you can stuff the pocket.)
- In fast-food restaurants, order single, regular, or junior-size sandwiches and stay away from the doubles and triples.
- Start the day without a serving of meat at breakfast.

Joaquin's Story

Joaquin is 68 years old and works as a technician for a local cable television company. His job is fairly inactive. Joaquin has had type 2 diabetes for about 18 years. It was his 50th birthday present. He has not taken great care of his diabetes, partly because he never felt bad with high blood glucose levels.

Now, however, he is suffering the consequences. Joaquin just found out he has some initial signs of diabetes kidney disease, including a small amount of protein in his urine (microalbuminuria). Joaquin's doctor advised him to speak with a dietitian about making changes in what he eats to lower his blood glucose, get his blood pressure under control, and help delay further kidney damage. Joaquin was concerned and quickly made an appointment with the dietitian.

The RD started by asking Joaquin what he usually eats. She asked him to be as honest as possible. She quickly found that Joaquin eats a lot of meat. Joaquin typically eats two large servings of meat each day. Lunch is often a large Italian submarine sandwich, a double cheeseburger, or a mile-high corned beef sandwich from a local sandwich shop. These choices present two problems. One is the large portion of meat, and the other is the high sodium count in these restaurant choices. Joaquin usually eats dinner at home, and the center of his plate is occupied by 6 or more ounces of chicken breast, hamburger, or pork chops or several pieces of fried fish.

Because Joaquin eats a lot of meat and he has the beginning signs of kidney disease, the dietitian decided to focus her teaching and suggestions on encouraging Joaquin to eat smaller amounts of meats that contain less sodium than his current choices. First, the RD made Joaquin aware that he eats much more meat than his body needs, particularly now that he has kidney damage. She added that Joaquin can help delay the progression of his kidney disease by keeping his blood glucose and blood pressure on target with medications, as well as by eating less sodium and protein. The dietitian gave Joaquin a few suggestions for cutting back on the amount of meat he eats.

(continues)

Joaquin's Story *(continued)*

Here are some of the lunch ideas the RD suggested:

- In a sub shop, order a small sub with turkey, smoked turkey, or roast beef. Hold the mayonnaise and oil and ask for mustard and plenty of lettuce, tomatoes, and onions.
- In a fast-food spot, order a single hamburger or grilled chicken sandwich and fill up on a baked potato or a garden salad with a small amount of light dressing.

For dinner, the RD suggested that Joaquin purchase a small food scale so that he can see how much meat he currently eats. She recommended that he try to eat no more than 3 to 4 ounces of cooked meat at dinner. He could make pasta, potatoes, rice, and other starches a bigger part of his dinner meal. He should try to get at least two vegetables or a double serving of one at dinner as well. As Joaquin learns what 3 ounces looks like on a food scale and on his plate, he can eyeball the quantity he should eat when he is out for dinner and share or take home the extra.

Before he left, Joaquin made an appointment to return to see the RD in about three weeks. At that time, he will bring his blood glucose records with a list of the meals and snacks that he has eaten. They will discuss how he can reach his blood glucose goals and how he is doing with the new ways to eat less meat and lower-sodium types of meats.

Serving Sizes for Meat and Meat Substitutes

Food	Serving Size	Calories	Protein (g)	Fat (g)	Saturated Fat (g)	Cholesterol (mg)
LEAN MEATS						
Beef jerky, dried	0.5 oz	58	4.7	3.6	1.5	7
Beef tenderloin, lean, broiled	1 oz	55	8.1	2.2	0.8	22
Beef, chipped, dried	1 oz	47	8.2	1.1	0.0	12
Beef, chuck, pot roast, lean only, cooked	1 oz	61	9.3	2.3	0.9	29
Beef, cubed steak, lean, cooked	1 oz	57	8.9	2.2	0.7	27
Beef, flank steak, lean, cooked	1 oz	53	7.9	2.1	0.9	14
Beef, ground round, cooked	1 oz	57	10.3	1.4	0.5	26
Beef, rib roast, lean, roasted	1 oz	65	7.7	3.5	1.4	23
Beef, round steak, lean, cooked	1 oz	61	9.6	2.2	0.8	29
Beef, rump roast, cooked	1 oz	59	8.9	2.3	0.8	27
Beef, sirloin, lean, cooked	1 oz	52	8.6	1.6	0.6	16
Beef, top round, braised	1 oz	56	10.2	1.4	0.5	26
Buffalo (bison), roasted	1 oz	41	8.1	0.7	0.3	23
Canadian bacon, grilled	1 oz	52	6.9	2.4	0.8	16
Catfish fillet, cooked	1 oz	43	5.3	2.3	0.5	18

Cheese, American, fat-free	1 slice	30	5.0	0.0	0.0	3
Cheese, American, reduced-fat	1 oz	68	5.4	2.5	4.0	14
Cheese, cheddar, fat-free	1 oz	45	9.0	0.0	0.0	3
Cheese, feta, fat-free, plain	1 oz	30	6.0	0.0	0.0	0
Cheese, mozzarella, fat-free	1 oz	45	7.9	0.0	0.0	4
Cheese, ricotta, fat-free	1/4 cup	45	8.0	0.0	0.0	20
Cheese, swiss, fat free	1 oz	41	6.8	0.0	0.0	7
Chicken breast, meat only, cooked	1 oz	47	8.8	1.0	0.3	24
Chicken, dark meat, no skin, roasted	1 oz	58	7.7	2.8	0.8	26
Clams, fresh, cooked	1 oz	42	7.2	0.6	0.1	19
Cod fillet, cooked	1 oz	30	6.5	0.2	0.0	16
Cornish game hen, cooked, no skin	1 oz	38	6.6	1.1	0.3	30
Cottage cheese, creamed, 4.5% milkfat	1/4 cup	54	6.5	2.3	1.0	8
Cottage cheese, low-fat, 1% milkfat	1/4 cup	41	7.0	0.6	0.4	2
Cottage cheese, nonfat	1/4 cup	40	7.0	0.0	0.0	3
Crab, steamed	1 oz	29	5.7	0.5	0.1	28
Duck, domestic, no skin, roasted	1 oz	57	6.6	3.2	1.0	25
Egg substitute (Egg Beaters)	1/4 cup	30	6.0	0.0	0.0	0

(continues)

Adapted from *Choose Your Foods: Exchange Lists for Diabetes* (American Dietetic Association and American Diabetes Association, 2008).

Serving Sizes for Meat and Meat Substitutes (continued)

Food	Serving Size	Calories	Protein (g)	Fat (g)	Saturated Fat (g)	Cholesterol (mg)
Egg white	2 egg whites	33	6.9	0.0	0.0	0
Flounder, cooked	1 oz	33	6.8	0.4	0.1	19
Goose, no skin, roasted	1 oz	67	8.2	3.6	1.0	27
Haddock, cooked	1 oz	32	6.9	0.3	0.0	21
Halibut fillet, cooked	1 oz	40	7.6	0.8	0.1	12
Ham, boiled lean deli, sandwich type (≤3 g fat/oz)	1 oz	29	4.5	1.0	0.5	15
Ham, canned, fully cooked	1 oz	64	5.8	4.3	1.4	18
Ham, cured, roasted	1 oz	44	7.1	1.6	0.5	16
Ham, extra lean (95% fat free)	1 oz	30	4.5	1.0	0.4	14
Heart, beef, cooked	1 oz	50	8.1	1.6	0.0	55
Herring, smoked	1 oz	61	7.0	3.5	1.0	23
Hot dog or frankfurter, (≤3 g fat/oz)	1 frankfurter	70	6.0	2.5	1.0	20
Kidney, beef, cooked	1 oz	45	7.7	1.3	0.3	203
Lamb leg, sirloin, roast, lean	1 oz	58	8.0	2.6	0.9	26
Lamb loin, roast or chop, cooked	1 oz	61	8.5	2.8	1.0	27
Liver, chicken, cooked	1 oz	47	6.9	1.8	0.6	159

Food	Serving				
Lobster, fresh, steamed	1 oz	28	5.8	0.2	0.0	20
Lox (smoked salmon)	1 oz	33	5.2	1.2	0.3	6
Orange roughy, cooked, dry heat	1 oz	30	6.4	0.3	0.0	23
Ostrich, cooked	1 oz	40	7.6	0.8	0.0	27
Oysters, cooked	6 medium	46	4.1	1.2	0.4	22
Pork chop, cooked	1 oz	57	8.4	2.4	0.9	24
Pork tenderloin, cooked	1 oz	40	7.4	1.0	0.3	21
Rabbit, cooked	1 oz	58	8.6	2.4	0.7	24
Salmon, canned, solids and liquids	1 oz	39	5.6	1.7	0.4	16
Salmon, fresh, broiled or baked	1 oz	61	7.7	3.1	0.5	25
Sardines, packed in oil, drained	2 small (2 2/3" x 1/2" x 1/4")	50	5.9	2.7	0.4	34
Sausage, smoked, (≤3 g fat/oz)	1 oz	40	3.5	1.3	0.5	12
Scallops, fresh steamed	1 oz	32	6.6	0.4	0.0	15
Shellfish, imitation	1 oz	29	3.4	0.4	0.0	6
Shrimp, fresh, cooked in water	1 oz	28	5.9	0.3	0.1	55
Steak, porterhouse, lean, broiled	1 oz	60	7.5	3.1	1.1	19
Steak, t-bone, lean, broiled	1 oz	57	7.6	2.8	1.0	16
Tilapia fillet, cooked	1 oz	37	7.4	0.8	0.3	25

(continues)

Adapted from *Choose Your Foods: Exchange Lists for Diabetes* (American Dietetic Association and American Diabetes Association, 2008).

Serving Sizes for Meat and Meat Substitutes (continued)

Food	Serving Size	Calories	Protein (g)	Fat (g)	Saturated Fat (g)	Cholesterol (mg)
Trout, cooked	1 oz	54	7.5	2.4	0.4	21
Tuna, canned in oil, drained	1 oz	53	7.5	2.3	0.0	9
Tuna, canned in water, drained	1 oz	33	7.2	0.2	0.1	8
Tuna, fresh, cooked	1 oz	52	8.5	1.8	0.5	14
Turkey breast (cutlet), no skin, roasted	1 oz	38	8.5	0.2	0.1	23
Turkey ham (≤3 g fat/oz)	1 oz	36	5.4	1.4	0.0	16
Turkey kielbasa (≤3 g fat/oz)	1 oz	45	4.0	2.5	1.0	16
Turkey pastrami (≤ 3 g fat/oz)	1 oz	40	5.2	1.8	1.0	15
Turkey, dark meat, no skin, cooked	1 oz	53	8.1	2.0	1.0	24
Veal loin, chop, cooked	1 oz	64	9.5	2.6	0.7	35
Veal roast	1 oz	55	9.0	1.9	0.5	33
Venison (deer), roast	1 oz	45	8.5	0.9	0.4	32
MEDIUM FAT MEATS						
Beef patty, ground, extra lean, pan broil (85% lean)	1 oz	66	7.0	4.0	1.6	24
Beef patty, ground, lean, pan broiled (80% lean)	1 oz	68	6.8	4.5	1.7	24
Beef patty, ground, regular, pan broiled (75% lean)	1 oz	70	6.6	4.7	1.8	23

Beef, prime rib, roasted	1 oz	83	7.7	5.5	2.4	23
Beef, shortribs, cooked	1 oz	84	8.7	5.1	2.2	26
Cheese spread	1 oz	82	4.6	6.0	3.8	16
Cheese, colby jack, reduced-fat	1 oz	80	7.0	5.0	3.5	15
Cheese, feta, regular	1 oz	75	4.0	6.0	4.2	25
Cheese, Mexican, reduced-fat	1 oz	81	8.1	6.0	3.0	20
Cheese, Monterey jack, reduced-fat	1 oz	80	7.0	6.0	3.5	20
Cheese, mozzarella (part skim milk)	1 oz	72	6.9	4.5	2.9	18
Cheese, mozzarella, reduced-fat	1 oz	70	8.0	4.0	2.5	15
Cheese, ricotta (part skim milk)	1/4 cup	85	7.0	4.9	3.0	19
Cheese, string	1 oz	83	7.1	5.3	3.5	18
Cheese, Swiss, reduced-fat	1 oz	70	9.0	3.5	2.0	10
Chicken, with skin, roasted	1 oz	68	7.7	3.8	1.1	25
Chicken, meat and skin, fried, flour coated	1 oz	76	8.1	4.2	1.1	25
Corned beef brisket, cooked	1 oz	71	5.1	5.4	1.8	28
Dove, cooked	1 oz	62	6.8	3.7	1.1	33
Duck, wild, meat and skin, (not cooked)	1 oz	60	4.9	4.3	1.4	23
Egg, fresh	1 egg	74	6.3	5.0	1.5	212

(continues)

Adapted from *Choose Your Foods: Exchange Lists for Diabetes* (American Dietetic Association and American Diabetes Association, 2008).

Serving Sizes for Meat and Meat Substitutes (continued)

Food	Serving Size	Calories	Protein (g)	Fat (g)	Saturated Fat (g)	Cholesterol (mg)
Fish, fried, cornmeal coating	1 oz	65	5.1	3.8	1.0	23
Goose, wild, with skin, cooked	1 oz	86	7.1	6.2	1.9	26
Lamb rib, roasted	1 oz	66	7.4	3.8	1.3	25
Lamb, ground, broiled	1 oz	80	7.0	5.6	2.3	27
Meatloaf	1 oz	65	6.0	3.9	1.5	17
Pheasant (grouse), cooked, meat and skin	1 oz	70	9.2	3.4	1.0	25
Pork cutlet, cooked	1 oz	71	7.9	4.2	1.5	24
Pork, Boston blade, roasted	1 oz	76	6.5	5.3	2.0	24
Sausage, hard (<5 g fat/oz)	1 oz	45	4.0	2.5	1.0	15
Tongue (beef), cooked	1 oz	80	5.5	6.3	2.3	37
Turkey, ground, cooked	1 oz	67	7.7	3.7	1.0	29
Veal cutlet, lean, cooked	1 oz	57	10.4	1.4	0.5	38
HIGH FAT MEATS						
Bacon, fried, drained	2 slices (16 per lb)	85	5.9	6.6	2.2	17
Bacon, turkey	3 slices	92	7.1	6.7	2.0	24

Bologna	1 oz	90	3.3	8.0	3.0	16
Cheese, American	1 oz	106	6.3	8.9	5.6	27
Cheese, blue-veined (blue, Roquefort)	1 oz	100	6.1	8.2	5.0	21
Cheese, cheddar-type	1 oz	114	7.1	9.4	6.0	30
Cheese, goat, hard	1 oz	127	8.6	10.0	6.9	30
Cheese, Monterey jack	1 oz	106	7.0	8.6	5.0	25
Cheese, Swiss, regular	1 oz	108	7.6	7.9	5.0	26
Chorizo sausage, Mexican or Spanish, cooked	1 oz	95	3.5	8.5	3.0	20
Hot dog (weiner, frankfurter)	1 hot dog (10/lb)	137	5.2	12.4	4.8	22
Hot dog, chicken	1 hot dog (10/lb)	116	5.8	8.8	2.5	45
Hot dog, turkey	1 hot dog (10/lb)	102	6.4	8.0	2.7	48
Pastrami, regular	1 oz	99	4.9	8.3	3.0	26
Pork sausage, cooked	1 oz	104	5.6	8.8	3.1	23
Pork spareribs, cooked, lean & fat	1 oz	112	8.2	8.6	3.2	34
Pork, ground, cooked	1 oz	84	7.3	5.9	2.2	27
Queso asadero (Mexican melting cheese)	1 oz	101	6.4	8.0	5.1	30
Salami, hard	1 oz	105	7.4	8.2	3.1	28
Sausage, bratwurst, fresh, cooked	1 oz	97	4.7	7.4	2.7	19

(continues)

Adapted from *Choose Your Foods: Exchange Lists for Diabetes* (American Dietetic Association and American Diabetes Association, 2008).

Serving Sizes for Meat and Meat Substitutes (continued)

Food	Serving Size	Calories	Protein (g)	Fat (g)	Saturated Fat (g)	Cholesterol (mg)
Sausage, Italian, cooked	1 oz	91	5.7	7.3	3.0	22
Sausage, knockwurst, cooked	1 oz	87	3.4	7.9	3.0	16
Sausage, Polish	1 oz	92	4.0	8.1	3.0	20
Sausage, smoked	1 oz	91	3.4	8.1	2.8	16
Sausage, summer	1 oz	95	4.5	8.4	3.0	21
PLANT-BASED PROTEINS (FOR BEANS, PEAS, AND LENTILS SEE STARCH LIST)						
Almond butter, plain	1 tbsp	91	2.9	8.6	0.8	0
"Bacon" strips, soy-based	3 strips	68	9.0	3.0	0.0	0
Breakfast patty, meatless (soy-based)	1 patty (1 1/2 oz)	79	9.9	2.8	0.5	0
Cashew butter, plain	1 tbsp	86	2.6	7.2	1.2	0
"Chicken" nuggets, breaded (soy-based)	2 nuggets (1 1/2 oz)	90	7.0	3.5	0.5	0
Edamame	1/2 cup	95	8.4	4.0	0.5	0

Food	Serving					
Falafel (spiced chickpea and wheat)	3 patties (approx 2 1/4")	170	6.8	9.1	1.2	0
Frankfurter (hot dog), meatless (soy based)	1 frankfurter (1 1/2 oz)	70	8.0	2.0	0.0	0
Hummus	1/3 cup	137	6.5	7.9	1.2	0
Meatless burger (soy-based)	1 patty (3 oz)	117	12.0	5.0	0.6	0
Meatless burger (vegetable- and starch-based)	1 patty	130	13.0	3.0	1.0	15
Meatless "beef" crumbles (soy-based)	2 oz	60	13.0	0.5	0.1	0
Meatless "sausage" crumbles (soy-based)	2 oz	60	7.0	0.0	0.0	0
Peanut butter, smooth or crunchy	1 tbsp	96	4.0	8.4	1.6	0
Soy nut butter	1 tbsp	96	4.4	8.0	1.0	0
Soy nuts, dry roasted, no salt	3/4 oz	96	8.4	4.6	0.7	0
Tempeh (bean cake)	1/4 cup	84	8.0	3.2	0.0	0
Tofu, firm	4 oz (1/2 cup)	80	9.3	4.7	1.0	0
Tofu, lite, firm, silken	4 oz (1/2 cup)	45	7.5	1.5	0.2	0

Adapted from *Choose Your Foods: Exchange Lists for Diabetes* (American Dietetic Association and American Diabetes Association, 2008).

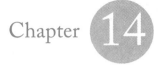

Fats and Oils

What You'll Learn:

- the foods in the fats group and their nutrition assets and liabilities
- healthy eating goals for fats and oils
- a frame of reference for how much fat most people eat
- questions to ask to get to know your current habits
- the number of servings of fats to eat based on your calorie needs
- the different types of fats, how they affect your blood lipid levels, and how to eat the right amounts of them
- tips to help you choose and use healthier fats and oils
- how to figure your total and saturated fat intake
- how to choose and use fat-free foods
- tips for slimming down your favorite recipes
- the serving sizes and nutrition numbers for fats

Foods in the Fats Group

The foods in this group include mainly the fats and oils that you use when you prepare or eat foods. They also include a small number of foods that provide most of their calories as fat. Some are healthier, like nuts, peanut butter, avocado, and seeds, and some are not so healthy, like bacon and sausage. This group doesn't include the fat that is part of meat or cheese. This fat is factored into your choices from the meat and meat substitute group.

Nutrition Assets of Fat

Fat is essential for keeping your body healthy. You need two essential fats, or more precisely, fatty acids—linoleic acid and alpha linolenic acid—because your body can't make them from other fats. These fatty acids are widely available in foods, and most people have no problem getting enough of them. Fat in foods is in the form of triglycerides—three fatty acid chains with a glycerol molecule. When you eat fats, they are broken down into glycerol and fatty acids. The body uses them to form nonessential fatty acids. Fat is stored in the body as triglycerides.

Fats are carriers for the fat-soluble vitamins A, D, E, and K and for carotenoids, which are essential to health. Fats are also important for maintaining healthy skin, and they become part of some of your body's hormones. Fat provides a source of energy when your primary source of energy, carbohydrate, runs out. (See chapter 7 for information on the best foods to eat to make sure you get enough vitamins and minerals.)

Saturated or Unsaturated

Fats and oils are divided into two main types: saturated and unsaturated. Unsaturated fats may be either polyunsaturated or monounsaturated. Omega-3 fats, which are present in some fattier fish, flax, walnuts, and some oils and appear to have benefits in lowering triglycerides, are in the category of polyunsaturated fats. All fats, from margarine to beef fat and canola oil, are made from varying amounts of these different types of fats or fatty acids. Most foods that contain fat contain varying amounts of saturated and unsaturated fats. Foods that contain a lot of saturated fats come from animal sources—butter, whole milk, and meats—as well as some oils, such as coconut and palm kernel oil. Animal sources of fat may also contain cholesterol. Foods that contain mainly unsaturated fats, such as corn or soybean oil, are from non-animal sources. (See pages 189–194 for more information on types of fat.)

The different fats and oils you eat have different effects on your blood lipids—your total blood cholesterol, LDL (bad cholesterol), HDL (good cholesterol), and triglycerides. (Chapter 1 describes the ADA blood lipid goals.) The fats that contain the most unsaturated fats (polyunsaturated and monounsaturated) are the healthiest. These tend to be in the liquid oils you eat. Saturated fat and trans fat are the least healthy. They even seem to cause an increase in insulin resistance. Saturated and trans fats tend to be the solid fats you eat.

Fat: Added or Attached?

To see how the fat grams creep into your meals, you can divide them into two categories: "added fats" and "attached fats." Added fats are fats that you use to prepare and eat food—the oil to fry an egg, the mayonnaise in seafood salad, salad dressing on salad, cream cheese on bagels, sour cream on baked potatoes, and cream in a cream sauce or soup. Find ways to cut down on these fats and oils.

In foods with attached fats, the fat is simply part of the food. For example, there is no way to take the fat out of nuts, peanut butter, eggs, prime rib, or avocado. The fat is attached and there to stay. The way to reduce the amount of fat you get from these foods is to eat less of them or avoid them altogether.

Fat Calories Add Up

Along with flavor, fat adds calories. Fat contains nine calories per fat gram—more than twice as many as the four calories per gram for carbohydrate and protein. Fat comes in small, calorie-dense packages.

Nutritional Value of Foods with and without Added Fat

Food	Serving	Calories	Fat (g)	Sat. Fat (g)	Chol. (mg)
Bread	1 slice	65	1	0	0
Bread with 1 tsp butter	1 slice	100	5	2	10
Bread with 1 tsp margarine	1 slice	100	5	1	0
Macaroni	1 cup	197	1	0	0
Macaroni and cheese	1 cup	430	22	9	42
Chicken breast, roasted, no skin	3 oz	142	3	1	72
Chicken breast, roasted, with skin	3 oz	165	7	2	71
Chicken breast, fried, with skin	3 oz	218	11	3	71

That's a big problem. The other is that eating fats from animal sources adds saturated fat and cholesterol to your meals.

Fat Adds Taste

Why is fat in so many foods? The answer is simple: fat makes food taste good, and Americans have gotten used to that flavor. Fats make you feel full. Fats also hold moisture in foods like baked goods and create the creamy texture of mayonnaise and salad dressings. Because fat plays so many roles in foods, it is difficult to make a great-tasting low-fat or fat-free food; however, today there are plenty of good-tasting lower-fat foods than ever before.

Fats: How People Eat

On average, Americans eat just under 35% of their calories as fat. That's on the high end of the recommended range of 20 to 35%, but not extremely high. The big problem is not the total amount of fat, it's the saturated fat and cholesterol in foods. Most Americans eat slightly less than 300 milligrams of cholesterol a day. Far and away the biggest cause for concern is the higher than desirable consumption of saturated fat. Excess amounts of saturated fat are related to high LDL (bad cholesterol) and an increased risk of heart and blood vessel problems. Given the amount of red meat, full-fat milk and cheese, ice cream, desserts, and fried restaurant foods we eat, it's no surprise that saturated fat intake is too high. Trans fat, which mainly comes from processed foods that contain partially hydrogenated fat, is also a cause for concern. We don't eat that much trans fat, and it's easier to eat even less now that manufacturers have started to decrease trans fat in their products. Nutrition experts agree that it's best to get trans fat down as low as possible.

Get to Know Yourself

If you want to change your eating habits, you need to know what you eat now. Ask yourself these questions about fats:

- Which fats and oils do I have in the refrigerator and cupboards?
- Can I buy and use healthier oils and cut down on unhealthy fats and oils?
- How much fat and oil do I use each day in food preparation, in and on foods I eat, and from restaurant foods?
- How often do I eat fried foods?
- What low-fat and fat-free foods do I buy to reduce the amount of fat I eat?
- When I eat in restaurants, do I attempt to minimize the amount of fat I eat by ordering lower fat items and limited added fats from salad dressing, sour cream, butter, etc.?

How Many Servings of Fats for You?

In chapter 6 you determined that a certain calorie range was the best for you. Find that calorie range in the chart on page 187 and then spot the number of servings of fats and oils you need each day. It is somewhere between 6 and 12.

Each fat serving has about 5 g of fat and 45 calories. The chart on pages 204–209 at the end of the chapter shows the serving sizes for added fats, along with information on their calories, total fat, type of fats, and cholesterol content. The foods in the chart are divided into groups by the fat they have the most of—saturated, polyunsaturated, and monounsaturated. Because the calories from fat add up very quickly, it is particularly important to pay attention to serving sizes. An extra teaspoon of regular margarine or butter adds 50 calories and an extra tablespoon of creamy dressing can be an extra 70 or more calories.

> ● QUICK TIP
>
> Your eyes can deceive you when it comes to fat content in a food. Measure fats as often as possible to make sure your eyes are still estimating correctly.

Sample Meal Plan

The sample meal plan on page 188 gives you an idea of how to fit six servings of fat into your day. The sample is designed for a person who needs 1,400–1,600 calories a day. Chapter 6 provides sample plans for other calorie ranges, along with nutritional information for several plans.

Fats and Diabetes

If you have diabetes, you are at risk for, or may already have, high blood pressure and/or abnormal blood lipids. Because of the strong connection between diabetes and heart and blood vessel disease, it's important to keep the amount of saturated fat you eat to less than 7% of your calories. You'll want to be extra vigilant about keeping the amount of saturated and trans fat you eat to a minimum and using the healthiest oils for cooking and eating.

Find Your Calorie Range

Which category fits you?	Women who... • want to lose weight • are small in size • and/or are sedentary	Women who... • are older and smaller • are larger and want to lose weight • and/or are sedentary	Women who... • are moderate to large size Men who... • are older • are small to moderate size and want to lose weight	Children Teen girls Women who... • are larger size and active Men who... • are small to moderate size and are at desired body weight	Teen boys Men who... • are active and moderate to large size
Daily calorie range	1,200–1,400	1,400–1,600	1,600–1,900	1,900–2,300	2,300–2,800
How Many Servings of Fats Do You Need Each Day?					
Fats	6	6	8	9	12

One-Day Meal Plan: 1,400–1,600 Calories

BREAKFAST

1/2 whole grain bagel (2 oz) with	2 starches
1 1/2 Tbsp light cream cheese	**1 fat**
3/4 cup blueberries with	1 fruit
1/3 cup plain fat-free yogurt	1/2 milk

LUNCH

Tuna salad made with	
2 oz tuna (1/2 cup), water-packed	2 oz meat
1 Tbsp light mayonnaise	**1 fat**
2 Tbsp diced celery	1 vegetable
1 Tbsp diced onions	
Tomato slices	
2 slices whole-wheat bread	2 starches
1 cup raw or blanched broccoli	1 vegetable
1 cup fat-free milk	1 milk
1/2 large apple	1 fruit

DINNER

3 oz grilled salmon with	3 oz meat
lemon and herbs	free food
Stir-fried vegetables with	
1/4 cup onions, cooked	2 vegetables
1/2 cup snow peas, cooked	
1/2 cup red peppers, cooked	
2 tsp canola oil	**2 fats**
1 cup brown rice	3 starches

EVENING SNACK

Mix together:	
1/2 cup crushed canned pineapple	1 fruit
(packed in own juice)	
1/3 cup plain fat-free yogurt	1/2 milk
1/8 cup chopped pecans	**2 fats**

Choosing unsaturated oils—ones with mainly monounsaturated and polyunsaturated fat—will help you decrease your saturated fat intake and lower your LDL (bad cholesterol). As for dietary cholesterol, keep it to no more than 200 milligrams each day. (For more information about the amount of fat you need when you have diabetes, see chapter 4.)

Today, nutrition experts agree that your main focus should be on choosing and eating healthy fats. Your secondary focus should be on eating less total fat, especially if you believe you eat more than 35% of your calories as fat. Learn more about the different types of fats in foods, and then use the suggestions provided on pages 190–194 to find out how you can eat more healthy unsaturated fats and fewer saturated and trans fats.

How the Fats You Eat Affect the Fats in Your Blood

Is It Healthy?	Type of Fat in Foods	Effect on Blood Lipids
Unhealthy fat	Saturated fat	↑ total cholesterol
		↑ LDL cholesterol
	Trans fat	↑ total cholesterol
		↑ LDL cholesterol
Healthy fat	Polyunsaturated fat	↓ total cholesterol
		↓ LDL cholesterol
		↓ HDL cholesterol
	Monounsaturated	↓ total cholesterol
		↓ LDL cholesterol
		↑ HDL cholesterol

Healthy Fats

Nutrition experts recommend that you get most of your calories from fat as a combination of polyunsaturated and monounsaturated fats. The chart above shows how these fats positively affect your blood lipids. See below to find out how you can get most of your fat calories from these healthier oils.

Polyunsaturated Fats

The two main types of polyunsaturated fats are the omega-3 fats and omega-6 fats. Both are good for your heart and blood lipids. Liquid vegetable oils, such as corn, soybean, and sunflower oils, contain mainly omega-6 polyunsaturated fats. Omega-3 fats are found in both plant and animal fats. The plant sources of omega-3 fats are canola and soybean oil, flax oil or seeds, and walnut oil or walnuts. Omega-3 fats are also contained in some fattier fish, such as salmon, trout, albacore tuna, and mackerel. Seafood contains more polyunsaturated fat in general than red meats and full-fat dairy foods do. Try to eat fish at least two times a week. Omega-3 polyunsaturated fats have been shown to lower triglycerides and decrease the "stickiness" of blood platelets, so that they don't stick to your artery walls.

Tips to Eat More Omega-6 Fats

- Choose processed foods made with healthier oils that aren't partially hydrogenated (trans).
- Use healthier oils in cooking, and use these instead of solid fat whenever possible. For example, scramble an egg in oil rather than with margarine.
- Choose a commercial salad dressing made with a healthy oil by reading the ingredient list. Most dressings are made with soybean oil. To cut calories, choose a low-fat, light, reduced-calorie, or fat-free salad dressing that has a taste you enjoy. Better yet, make your own salad dressing with a healthy oil. It can be much lower in sodium. Whatever salad dressing you use, pour cautiously.

Tips to Eat More Omega-3 Fats

- Eat fattier fish at least two times a week—salmon, trout, albacore tuna, sardines, eel, herring, and mackerel.
- Sprinkle ground flax seed on dry or cooked cereal, in casseroles, or on salads.
- Eat more walnuts or use walnut oil. Enjoy a small handful of walnuts as a snack or make a homemade salad dressing with walnut oil.

Monounsaturated Fats

Monounsaturated fats are good for your heart. The foods and oils that are the best sources of monounsaturated fats are nuts (other than walnuts and chestnuts); canola, olive, and peanut oil; olives; and avocados. The slight benefit of monounsaturated fats over polyunsaturated fats is that they may be able to raise your HDL (good cholesterol) level, whereas polyunsaturated fats seem to lower HDL while also lowering LDL. Research shows that they may also decrease insulin resistance.

Tips to Eat More Monounsaturated Fats

- Stock canola, olive, or a diacylglycerol (DAG) oil in your cupboard. Use them to sauté, cook, and bake (don't use olive oil for baked goods).
- Make your own salad dressing with canola or olive oil.
- Enjoy a handful of almonds, pecans, peanuts, cashews, or macadamia nuts as a snack. Sprinkle a few nuts onto salads, cooked or dry cereal, or stir-frys.
- Use a slice or two of avocado on a salad or sandwich. Garnish casseroles with avocado or use it to make guacamole.
- Add a few olives to a relish plate, toss them into a salad, or use as a garnish.

Unhealthy Fats

Saturated Fats

Foods with saturated fat are mainly from animal sources. Red meats, poultry, seafood, whole milk, cheese, ice cream, and butter all contain some saturated fat. Another group of foods—coconut, palm, and palm kernel oils—are used in some processed crackers, cookies, baked goods, and fried snack foods. Check the chart on page 189 to see what saturated fats do to your blood lipids.

Tips to Cut Down on Saturated Fat

- Purchase lean cuts of meat and trim the visible fat before cooking.
- Take the skin off poultry (either before or after cooking).
- Eat smaller portions (3 oz cooked) of meat and meat substitutes. Prepare them in low-fat ways.
- Limit the amount of full-fat cheese you eat, and buy reduced-fat and part-skim cheeses.
- Use fat-free and low-fat dairy foods such as milk and yogurt.
- Try different brands of low-fat, light, or fat-free cream cheese, cottage cheese, mayonnaise, and sour cream. See if any of them satisfy your palate and needs.
- Opt for a heart-healthy liquid oil or tub margarine instead of using butter, shortening, or other solid fats for cooking and eating.
- Limit the amount of coconut, palm, and palm kernel oil you eat. They are saturated fats in processed foods. Check the ingredient list for these fats.

Trans Fats

About 80% of the trans fats Americans eat are from processed foods that contain partially hydrogenated oils. Only about 20% of trans fats are from foods of animal origin, such as meats and dairy foods. The trans fats in processed foods are created through hydrogenation, a process that makes fat hard at room temperature and helps food stay fresh on supermarket shelves and in your cupboard. During hydrogenation, some of the healthy unsaturated fat becomes trans fat. For example, oil is hydrogenated to make margarine that is hard enough to form into sticks. In the last decade, research has linked trans fats to increased total and LDL cholesterol levels and, therefore, increased risk of heart disease.

Although we eat only about 3% of calories as trans fat, nutrition experts believe you'd be better off getting as little trans fats as possible. The best way to avoid trans fats is to avoid foods that contain partially hydrogenated fat as an ingredient in packaged foods. Keep in mind, though, that the best idea is still to reduce your saturated fat intake. When you reduce saturated fat, you'll automatically reduce trans fat. Since 2006, the FDA requires that most packaged foods have food labels stating the amount of trans fat they contain. This requirement has encouraged food manufacturers to get rid of some trans fats. Read more about food labels in chapter 22.

Tips for Cutting Down on Trans Fats

- Follow the tips for cutting down on saturated fat (see page 192). They will help you reduce your trans fats as well.
- Use the food label to check the amount of trans fats in packaged foods. Be aware of the serving size and keep in mind that manufacturers can list any amount of trans fat below 0.5 grams per serving as zero. Also read the ingredient list and try to limit foods that have partially hydrogenated oils among the top few ingredients.
- Choose a tub margarine or spread with little or no trans fat.
- Minimize the amount of fried restaurant foods you eat. The fat used for frying may contain trans fats.

Total Fat

Your nutrition goals for total fat will vary based on your current food choices. You may find that you don't eat too much fat, but you still need to work on choosing healthier fats. You may find that you need to work on both the amount and the type of fat you eat. The good news is that when you eat less total fat, you often also lower the amount of saturated and trans fats and cholesterol you eat.

The healthy eating plans in this book provide about 30% of calories as fat. You might find you want slightly more or less fat, but try to stick to between 25 and 35% of calories. You'll want to keep your saturated fat intake at no more than 7% of your calories on average. The remainder of your calories from fat should come from the healthier unsaturated fats.

Tips to Reduce Total Fat Intake

If you think you might be eating more than 35% of your calories as fat, try these tips for reducing your total fat intake:

- Use less butter, margarine, oil, salad dressing, mayonnaise, cheese, cream cheese, and sour cream. Take advantage of the reduced-fat and low-fat versions of these foods.
- Eat fried foods only once in a while (less than once a month).
- Prepare foods using low-fat methods—broiling, baking, braising, barbecuing, grilling, sautéing, and steaming.

Figure How Much Total Fat and Saturated Fat to Eat

Here's how to figure the amount of fat to eat each day. Suppose you're following an eating plan in which you eat 2,000 calories a day, and you want to get 30% of your calories from fat. To find 30% of 2,000 calories, multiply:

Total calories per day × *% of calories from fat* =
Daily calories from fat
2,000 calories × *30% (or .30)* = **600 calories from fat**

Because there are 9 calories in a gram of fat, you can find out how many grams of fat you need each day by dividing:

$$\frac{Daily\ calories\ from\ fat}{9\ calories\ per\ gram\ of\ fat} = \textbf{Daily grams of fat}$$
600 ÷ *9* = **67 grams of fat**

You can use these same calculations to figure how many grams of saturated fat to eat each day:

2,000 calories × *7% (or .07)* = **140 calories from
saturated fat**
140 ÷ *9* = **15 g of saturated fat**

Keep in mind that the 140 calories from saturated fat are part of the daily total of 600 calories from fat that you figured above, so, you can eat 67 grams of fat for the day, and no more than 14 grams of that number should come from saturated fat.

Cholesterol Facts

Cholesterol is actually not fat. In fact, two foods that are very high in cholesterol—liver and shrimp—are very low in fat. Another confusing point is that foods that are high in saturated fat are not necessarily high in cholesterol and vice versa. There is minimal difference between the cholesterol counts of lean meats and higher-fat meats. Cholesterol is discussed with fats because it is a fatlike substance that raises blood cholesterol. The diabetes guidelines encourage you to eat no more than 200 mg of cholesterol daily. Dietary cholesterol is found only in foods from animal sources—red meats, organ meats, poultry, seafood, egg yolk, and whole-milk dairy foods.

Tips to Cut Down on Cholesterol

- Eat smaller portions of red meat, poultry, and seafood.
- Choose reduced-fat and part-skim cheeses.
- Choose low-fat or fat-free milk and yogurt.
- Limit egg yolks to no more than 3 a week. Use egg whites or egg substitutes instead, or use a combination of one whole egg and one egg white when making scrambled eggs or omelets.
- Limit foods that are high in cholesterol, such as organ meats and shellfish.

Fat-Free Foods

Many of the ingredients that make fat-free foods possible are fat replacers. Most fat replacers in foods are made from carbohydrates. Their names are on thousands of ingredient lists—polydextrose, modified food starch, maltodextrins, hydrogenated starch hydrolysate, xanthan, and guar gum. Sometimes these fat replacers are made from corn or potato starch, simple sugars such as sucrose or corn syrup, or natural gums. Different fat replacers do different things in foods, so it is common to find several in one food.

Free Foods: Calories Add Up

Foods with fat replacers, low-calorie sweeteners, or sugar alcohols contain calories. Those calories come from the carbohydrate in the fat replacer as well as from other ingredients in the food. Consider the nutrition labels from a sugar-free and fat-free hot cocoa mix and fat-free mayonnaise:

Hot Cocoa

Nutrition Facts

Servings Size 1 envelope

Amount Per Serving

Calories 60	**Calories from Fat** 9

Total Fat 1 g
  Saturated Fat 0 g
  Trans Fat 0 g
Cholesterol 0 mg
Sodium 190 mg
Total Carbohydrate 10 g
  Dietary Fiber 1 g
  Sugars 6 g
Protein 2 g

Mayonnaise

Nutrition Facts

Serving Size 1 Tbsp

Amount Per Serving

Calories 25	**Calories from Fat** 9

Total Fat 1 g
  Saturated Fat 0 g
  Trans Fat 0 g
Cholesterol 0 mg
Sodium 140 mg
Total Carbohydrate 4 g
  Dietary Fiber 0 g
  Sugars 6 g
Protein 0 g

If you use several servings of fat-free or sugar-free foods in an average day, the calories can add up. Here's how to count the fat-free mayonnaise: 1 Tbsp = free; 2 Tbsp = 8 g carbohydrate. This adds up to one half of a starch serving.

Fat Replacers and Diabetes

When you have diabetes, you need to know what these carbohydrate-based fat replacers do to your blood glucose levels. If you substitute fat-free cream cheese that has no fat and some carbohydrate for regular cream cheese that has fat and very little carbohydrate, what is the effect on your blood glucose? Because carbohydrate raises blood glucose quicker and higher than fat, you might see a slight difference when you measure your blood glucose. Taste these foods and see how they affect your blood glucose. Then, consider your diabetes and nutrition goals and make a decision about whether they offer you benefits or not.

Counting Fat-Free Foods in Your Eating Plan

- A food or drink with fat replacers or low-calorie sweeteners that has 20 calories or less or 5 grams of carbohydrate or less in each serving is not likely to raise your blood glucose or add significant calories. These foods are free foods.

- Limit the use of fat-free foods with more than 20 calories or 5 grams of carbohydrate to three servings each day. Spread these servings out over the day.

- If a fat-free food has more than 20 calories and more than 5 grams of carbohydrate per serving, count it as part of your meal plan.

- If the calories are mainly from carbohydrate, count them as follows:
    6–10 g of carbohydrate counts as 1/2 starch, fruit, or milk serving (whichever fits the food).
    11–20 g of carbohydrate counts as 1 starch, fruit, or milk serving (whichever fits the food).

- If the calories are from fat, carbohydrate, and/or protein, use the directions in chapter 18 to figure out how to fit the food into your meal plan.

Tips for Slimming Down Your Favorite Recipes

Use the knowledge you gained about eating less fat to slim down your favorite recipes. What about Aunt Sally's macaroni and cheese recipe or Grandma Betty's apple cobbler? You may long for them, but they may be high in fat and calories from full-fat dairy foods, fats, and sweeteners.

- **Think of a recipe as a starting point.** Change it any way you want to make it tastier and healthier. For example, you might use a healthy oil rather than butter or margarine to sauté, use less oil to sauté, or add a few drizzles of cooking wine or sherry to add flavor without extra fat. Maybe you want to raise the fiber level of a meatloaf by adding bulgur or whole-wheat bread, or lower the saturated fat content by substituting ground turkey for a third of the meat, or increase the omega-3 content by adding a few teaspoons of ground flax. Increase the calcium content of an omelet by adding a tablespoon of nonfat dry milk to the egg mixture and coat the pan with a healthy oil instead of butter or margarine.
- **Keep in mind that it is easier to slim down recipes when you cook rather than when you bake.** You cannot make big changes in recipes for some baked items, such as chocolate cake or sponge cake, because there is a delicate chemistry between ingredients. In some fruit bread, pudding, cheesecake, and other recipes, however, you can cut the sugar by about a third and, if you need it to be sweeter, replace the sweetness with a low-calorie sweetener (sugar substitute) that can withstand heat.
- **Recipes that contain fruit, such as fruit cobbler, banana bread, carrot cake, or applesauce cake, will slim down, because fruit provides both sweetness and bulk (volume) to the recipe.** Lower the fat and calorie count of a pie by using a single bottom crust rather than top and bottom crusts. Look for similar recipes in low-calorie or diabetes cookbooks. Adapt your recipe or try theirs.
- **When you use less fat, you must add back flavor.** For flavor, add fat-free seasonings, spices, or herbs. Try new ones for new taste treats.
- **Use more or less of an ingredient.** For example, in a recipe for stir-fry, use less meat. Replace the volume with larger quantities of the vegetables in the recipe or add another vegetable, starch,

or fruit. For instance, add pineapple chunks and bean sprouts. A few drops of spicy hot oil add flavor with few calories.

- **In a meat sauce, use less meat and add more vegetables.** For example, sauté onions, peppers, mushrooms, and zucchini to add volume to the tomato sauce. In lasagna, use less meat and add a layer of spinach sautéed with a bit of oil and lots of garlic.

- **Substitute an ingredient with more flavor, such as extra-sharp cheese, so you can use less of it.** Or take advantage of lean but flavorful turkey sausage instead of using a larger amount of ground meat in a chili or soup.

- **Drain and pat dry ground meat, bacon, or sausage to get out as much excess fat as you can.**

- **Sauté with less oil or butter than the recipe calls for.** You might need to use a lower flame than suggested to avoid burning the food.

- **Skip the butter or margarine that is often called for in store-bought rice and grain mixtures.** They cook up just fine without it.

- **Take advantage of new reduced-fat and reduced-calorie ingredients in some recipes.** For example, you might want to top a Mexican dish with light or fat-free sour cream, make a dip with a combination of fat-free yogurt and light sour cream, or use light cream cheese to make a flavorful spread. Be careful when cooking or baking with these ingredients. When you melt margarine-like spreads that list water as the first ingredient, the water separates from the oil and splatters.

- **Use fresh herbs.** You can find them in the supermarket, but buy them no more than a few days before you cook so that they are fresh. If you do not use the fresh herb immediately, wrap it in a slightly damp paper towel, place it in a plastic bag, and use it within a few days. A less expensive way to have herbs is to grow them in a garden or pots. If your recipe calls for dried herbs, increase the amount of fresh herb you use by three.

- **Buy dry herbs and spices in small quantities because they lose taste over time.** If you use dry herbs instead of fresh, use only one-third the amount.

- **Check out recipe resources.** The Internet is loaded with recipes. www.diabetes.org is a good place to start. Borrow low-calorie and diabetes cookbooks and magazines from the library. Learn healthier ways of cooking and baking and gather recipes from television cooking shows.

Common Recipe Ingredients and Some Healthier Substitutes

Ingredient	Substitute
Bacon	Turkey bacon, Canadian bacon, smoked turkey, or lean ham
Butter, regular stick	Margarine or spread in a tub or a healthy oil
Cream cheese	Light, reduced-fat, or fat-free cream cheese
Mayonnaise	Reduced-calorie or fat-free mayonnaise, or mix regular mayonnaise with nonfat yogurt
Meat, ground	Extra-lean ground meat or ground turkey or a combination
Milk, whole	Fat-free milk, low-fat milk, or nonfat dry milk
Milk, evaporated	Fat-free evaporated milk
Sausage	Low-fat turkey sausage
Shortening	Healthy liquid oil
Sour cream	Light or nonfat sour cream, nonfat plain yogurt, or low-fat cottage cheese (puree in blender)

Anna's Story

Anna is a 57-year-old Latina woman who works as an administrative assistant for an insurance company. She recently found out that she has type 2 diabetes when she went to her nurse practitioner with symptoms of a yeast infection and blurred vision. The diabetes did not come as a surprise to Anna, because many people in her family have it. Anna is overweight by about 30 pounds. For several years, she has had high blood pressure for which she takes medication, and she tries to watch her salt and sodium intake. When her doctor diagnosed type 2 diabetes, he also found that Anna's blood lipids were abnormal.

Anna's nurse practitioner suggested she try to manage both her diabetes and her blood lipids with changes in her eating habits and some weight loss along with a low dose of the blood glucose–lowering drug metformin.

Anna was anxious to see a dietitian because she just was not feeling herself. The RD told Anna that it is common for people with type 2 diabetes who are overweight to also have high blood pressure and abnormal blood lipids. She stressed how important it is to keep these numbers on target to stay healthy. The best news Anna heard is that losing just a few pounds may improve her situation.

Anna listed what she usually eats. For breakfast during the week, Anna has a large muffin with margarine or a bagel with cream cheese and coffee. Weekend breakfasts are donuts, a cinnamon bun, or a cheese omelet along with toast and jam. She often eats lunch—tuna or chicken salad sandwich with chips and coleslaw—in the employee cafeteria. Sometimes she has fried chicken, mashed potatoes, and gravy with a green vegetable. Other times she goes out for a few slices of pizza with extra cheese and pepperoni or a hamburger and large French fries and regular soda.

Anna eats dinner at home and often has chicken or fish— fried because that is how her husband likes it. She tries to eat

(continues)

Anna's Story *(continued)*

one vegetable at dinner and adds margarine to that. She has two or three slices of bread with margarine at dinner. In the evening, she munches on cookies, chips, or ice cream.

The RD showed Anna that she eats too much meat and fat and too few vegetables, fruits, and milk. The first area Anna chose to work on was eating less fat. Together they developed a list of ways to lower fat, saturated fat, and cholesterol and to eat more healthy fats. For breakfast, Anna will bring a whole-wheat English muffin from home and use light or fat-free cream cheese or tub margarine and low-sugar jelly; if she has a muffin, she'll leave off the margarine. A breakfast of high-fiber cereal, fat-free milk, and fruit at home would be great. The RD suggested that Anna bring pieces of fruit to work to eat with lunch or as an afternoon snack.

For lunch, Anna would be better off choosing a plain meat sandwich—turkey, roast beef, and sometimes ham—rather than tuna or chicken salad. She can request mustard rather than mayonnaise and get more lettuce and tomato on top. A small bag of pretzels or popcorn, a small salad, or a cooked vegetable would be lower-fat side items. For hot meals, a vegetable plate, keeping fried items few and far between, would be healthy, as would a trip to the cafeteria salad bar. Pizza is fine as long as it is topped with vegetables rather than high-fat extra cheese and meats and she eats only two pieces rather than three or four.

At dinner, Anna should roast, grill, steam, or poach chicken or fish rather than fry it. Again, she should try to eat two servings of vegetables. Rather than putting margarine on top, Anna could add a squirt of lemon juice or a dash of a low-sodium herb combination. For evening snacks, Anna could try fat-free, sugar-free yogurt with fruit, cereal and fat-free milk, light popcorn, or a piece of fruit. Anna was willing to try these suggestions and to come back in several weeks.

Serving Sizes for Fats

Food	Serving Size	Calories	Fat (g)	Sat. Fat (g)	Mono-unsat. Fat (g)	Poly-unsat. Fat (g)	Cholesterol (mg)
MONOUNSATURATED FATS							
Almond butter, plain	1 1/2 tsps	45	4.3	0.4	2.8	0.9	0
Almonds, dry roasted	6 almonds	48	4.2	0.3	2.7	1.0	0
Avocado	2 tbsps	45	4.1	0.6	2.7	0.5	0
Brazil nuts	2 nuts	66	6.6	1.5	2.5	2.1	0
Cashew butter, plain	1 1/2 tsps	43	3.6	0.6	2.3	0.7	0
Cashews, salted	6 cashews	52	4.2	1.0	2.5	0.7	0
Hazelnuts (filberts)	5 nuts	45	4.4	0.3	3.3	0.6	0
Macadamia nuts, dry roasted, no salt added	3 nuts	56	5.9	0.9	4.6	0.1	0
Nuts, mixed	6 nuts	37	3.4	1.0	1.9	0.8	0
Oil, canola	1 tsp	40	4.5	0.3	2.7	1.3	0
Oil, olive	1 tsp	40	4.5	0.6	3.3	0.5	0
Oil, peanut	1 tsp	40	4.5	0.8	2.1	1.4	0
Olives, green, stuffed, large	10 olives	62	5.0	1.2	3.8	0.5	0
Olives, ripe (black), pitted	8 large	40	3.8	0.5	2.8	0.3	0

Peanut butter	1 1/2 tsps	48	4.2	0.8	2.0	1.2	0
Peanuts, dry roasted, no salt	10 peanuts	58	5.0	0.7	2.5	1.6	0
Pecans, dry roast	4 pecan halves	40	4.2	0.4	2.5	1.2	0
Pistachios	16 kernels	64	5.1	0.6	2.7	1.6	0
POLYUNSATURATED FATS						
Flaxseed, whole	1 tbsp	55	4.3	0.4	0.8	3.0	0
Margarine, liquid, regular	1 tsp	34	3.8	0.5	0.8	2.3	0
Margarine, regular, stick, 65–80% vegetable oil	1 tsp	30	3.3	0.7	0.9	1.0	0
Margarine, tub, 60–70% vegetable oil	1 tsp	24	2.7	0.6	0.9	1.1	0
Margarine-like spread, tub, light or lower-fat (30–50% vegetable oil)	1 tbsp	46	5.0	1.1	1.5	2.3	0
Mayonnaise	1 tsp	33	3.6	0.5	0.9	2.0	2
Mayonnaise, light (reduced fat)	1 tbsp	45	4.6	0.7	1.1	2.5	4
Mayonnaise-style salad dressing	2 tsps	27	2.3	0.3	0.7	1.3	3

(continues)

Adapted from *Choose Your Foods: Exchange Lists for Diabetes* (American Dietetic Association and American Diabetes Association, 2008).

Serving Sizes for Fats (continued)

Food	Serving Size	Calories	Fat (g)	Sat. Fat (g)	Mono- unsat. Fat (g)	Poly- unsat. Fat (g)	Cholesterol (mg)
Mayonnaise-style salad dressing, light	1 tbsp	25	1.5	0.3	0.2	1.0	4
Oil, corn	1 tsp	40	4.5	0.6	1.2	2.5	0
Oil, cottonseed	1 tsp	40	4.5	1.2	0.8	2.3	0
Oil, flaxseed	1 tsp	40	4.5	0.4	0.9	3.0	0
Oil, grapeseed	1 tsp	40	4.5	0.4	0.7	3.1	0
Oil, safflower	1 tsp	40	4.5	0.3	0.6	3.4	0
Oil, soybean	1 tsp	40	4.5	0.6	1.0	2.6	0
Oil, soybean and canola (Enova)	1 tsp	40	4.7	0.2	1.7	2.3	0
Oil, sunflower	1 tsp	40	4.5	0.5	0.9	3.0	0
Pine nuts (pignolia), dried	1 tbsp	58	5.9	0.4	1.6	2.9	0
Pumpkin seeds, roasted	1 tbsp	73	5.9	1.1	1.8	2.7	0
Salad dressing, reduced-fat, cream based	2 tbsps	70	4.0	0.3	1.8	1.5	0
Salad dressing, regular	1 tbsp	69	6.7	0.8	1.3	3.2	0
Sesame seeds	1 tbsp	52	4.5	0.6	1.7	2.0	0

Spread, plant stanol ester, light (Benecol)	1 tbsp	50	5.0	0.5	2.5	2.0	0
Spread, plant stanol ester, regular (Benecol)	2 tsps	47	5.0	0.3	1.7	1.3	0
Sunflower seeds, dry roasted	1 tbsp	47	4.0	0.4	0.8	2.6	0
Tahini (sesame butter or paste)	2 tsps	60	5.4	0.8	2.0	2.4	0
Walnuts, English, shelled	4 halves	52	5.2	0.5	0.7	3.8	0
SATURATED FATS							
Bacon grease	1 tsp	39	4.3	2.0	1.9	0.5	4
Bacon, fried, drained	1 slice (16 per lb)	43	3.3	1.1	1.5	0.4	9
Bacon, turkey	1 slice	31	2.2	0.7	0.9	0.5	8
Butter	1 tsp 5	3.8	2.4	0.0	10	1.0	27
Butter, light (Land O' Lakes)	1 tbsp	50	6.0	3.5	1.5	0.0	15
Butter, whipped	2 tsps	33	4.0	2.3	1.4	0.2	10
Butter blends with oil, light	1 tbsp	50	5.0	2.0	–	–	5
Butter blends with oil, regular	1 1/2 tsps	50	5.5	2.2	–	–	10
Chitterlings, boiled	2 tbsps (1/2 oz)	38	3.3	1.5	1.1	0.2	44
Coconut milk, light	1/3 cup	47	4.0	2.7	0.7	0.1	0
Coconut milk, regular	1 1/2 tbsps	44	4.8	4.3	0.2	0.1	0

(continues)

Adapted from *Choose Your Foods: Exchange Lists for Diabetes* (American Dietetic Association and American Diabetes Association, 2008).

Serving Sizes for Fats (continued)

Food	Serving Size	Calories	Fat (g)	Sat. Fat (g)	Mono-unsat. Fat (g)	Poly-unsat. Fat (g)	Cholesterol (mg)
Coconut, shredded, dried, sweetened	2 tbsps	42	2.6	2.4	0.1	0.0	0
Cream cheese	1 tbsp (1/2 oz)	51	4.6	3.1	1.4	0.2	20
Cream cheese, reduced-fat (neufchatel)	1 1/2 tbsps (3/4 oz)	54	4.6	3.1	1.5	0.2	15
Cream, half & half	2 tbsps	39	3.5	2.1	1.0	0.1	11
Cream, heavy (whipping, unwhipped)	1 tbsp	52	5.5	3.5	1.6	0.2	21
Cream, light	1 1/2 tbsps	44	4.3	2.7	1.3	0.2	15
Lard, pork	1 tsp	39	4.3	1.7	1.9	0.5	4

Oil, coconut	1 tsp	39	4.5	3.9	0.3	0.1	0
Oil, palm	1 tsp	40	4.5	2.2	1.7	0.4	0
Oil, palm kernel	1 tsp	39	4.5	3.7	0.5	0.1	0
Salt pork, fresh, cooked	1/4 oz	51	5.4	1.9	2.6	0.6	6
Shortening	1 tsp	38	4.3	1.1	1.9	1.1	0
Sour cream, reduced-fat or light	3 tbsps	61	3.7	3.0	0.6	0.2	18
Sour cream, regular	2 tbsps	62	4.8	3.4	1.4	0.1	19
Whipped cream, pressurized, regular	1/4 cup	39	3.3	2.1	1.0	0.1	11
Whipped cream, sweetened	2 tbsps	52	5.2	3.2	1.5	0.2	19

Adapted from *Choose Your Foods: Exchange Lists for Diabetes* (American Dietetic Association and American Diabetes Association, 2008).

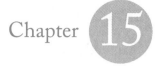
Sugars and Sweets

What You'll Learn:

- the foods in the sugars and sweets group
- the difference between the terms sugar and sugars
- the nutritional liabilities of sugars and sweets
- healthy eating goals for sugars
- a frame of reference for how much sweets people eat
- questions to ask yourself to get to know your current habits
- all about sugar alcohols, sugar substitutes, and sugar-free foods
- tips to help you keep added sugars and sweets to a bare minimum
- the serving sizes and nutrition numbers for sugars

Foods in the Sugars and Sweets Group

Sugars and sweets don't make up a food group, because you don't need sweets in a well-balanced eating plan. Sugars and sweets usually add calories that contain nearly no nutrients. Sugars can contribute a boatload of calories if you're not aware of how they creep into your foods (this is especially true of the calories in drinks). In other words, there are no particularly healthy or essential foods in this group. Are they enjoyable? Yes! Do you need to eliminate added sugars and sweets? No!

In this chapter, you'll learn how to keep added sugars to a minimum and how to fit in sweets in small quantities while you explore their effects on your blood glucose levels. You'll also determine how to make use of sugar substitutes and helpful sugar-free offerings from the supermarket.

What Are "Sugars"?

Notice the use of the term *sugars* instead of *sugar*. The term sugars does not refer just to the white granulated stuff, it more accurately describes two types of sugars in foods as follows:

- **Naturally occurring sugars:** Some healthy foods contain naturally occurring sugars, which provide healthy sources of energy, carbohydrate, vitamins, and minerals. Examples are the sucrose and fructose in fruit or the lactose in milk.
- **Added sugars:** The sugars added to foods during food processing, in food preparation, or at the table. Added sugars used in food manufacturing are now the greatest contributor of sugars to people's diet. Today, the most commonly added sugar is high fructose corn syrup.

All sugars—from natural sources or added—contain 4 calories per gram, because they are 100% carbohydrate. Knowing the various sugars helps you make decisions when you read Nutrition Facts labels.

What Are "Sweets"?

Sweets contain added sugars and they often contain fats. Think about cake, cookies, and ice cream. You may not realize that it's the fats in most sweets, not the sugars, that raise the calorie count. In addition, many sweets contain sources of saturated and trans fats and cholesterol depending on the ingredients used to make the sweets. If a sweet contains butter and eggs, it will contain cholesterol. If it contains partially hydrogenated fat, it will contain trans fat. If you need to lose weight or if you have problems with your blood fats, particularly triglycerides—and both are likely situations if you have pre-diabetes or type 2 diabetes—you need to cut back on sweets. The chart below shows how the calories mount up when fat creeps into desserts.

Nutritional Value of Some Desserts with and without Added Fat				
Food	Serving	Calories	Carb (g)	Fat (g)
Strawberry gelatin (regular)	1/2 cup	70	15	0
Strawberry pie (two-crust)	1 serving	360	49	18
Chocolate chips	1 Tbsp	66	9	4
Chocolate chip cookies	2 small	248	28	14
Jelly beans	10 (1 oz)	66	26	0
Lemon meringue pie	1 piece	362	49	16
Sugar, granulated	1 Tbsp	48	12	0
Ice cream (regular, store brand)	1/2 cup	132	16	7
Ice cream (premium)	1/2 cup	280	20	20

Sugars and Sweets: How Much People Eat

The consumption of added sugars is one of the greatest nutritional concerns today. The intake of added sugars has steadily risen over the last two decades. Many health experts believe that this extra sugar is a big contributor to the twin epidemics of obesity and type 2 diabetes, as well as a big reason people don't eat enough nutrient-dense foods. Americans eat an estimated 22 teaspoons of added sugars every day! Think about that pile of sugar. It sounds hard to believe, but when you consider that a 20-ounce regularly sweetened soft drink contains about 15 teaspoons of added sugars, it becomes much easier to believe. Beyond regularly sweetened soft drinks, which contribute over 30% of these added sugars, the other large sources of added sugars are in candy; cake, cookies, food bars, and pies; fruit drinks (like punch and sport drinks); and dairy desserts.

> ● **QUICK TIP**
>
> As you add up the amount of added sugars you eat, you may realize that one of the quickest and easiest ways to lose weight and scale back on carbohydrates is to change what you drink.

Recommendations for healthy eating suggest you eat no more than a few teaspoons of added sugars a day. The fewer calories you can eat, the less added sugars you can eat. The table below applies those guidelines to the calorie ranges listed in this book. As you can see, there isn't much room for added sugars or sweets.

Calorie Range	Sugars (tsp)
1,200–1,400	4
1,400–1,600	4
1,600–1,900	4–7
1,900–2,300	8–11
2,300–2,800	12–18

Get to Know Yourself

If you want to change your eating habits, you need to know what you eat now. Ask yourself these questions about sugars and sweets:

- Which foods and beverages do I add sugars to in preparation or at the table?
- Which foods do I eat that contain added sugars? How often and in what quantity do I eat these foods?
- Do I use sugar substitutes?
- How many times a day or a week do I eat sweets?
- What are my favorite sweets?
- How often do I need to eat sweets to stay on track with a healthy eating plan?

Sugars and Sweets and Diabetes

People with diabetes no longer have to avoid sugars and sweets. This has been the ADA recommendation since 1994. Today's diabetes nutrition guidelines point out that similar amounts of carbohydrate from all sources of carbohydrate—bread, pasta, fruit, or sugar from sweets—raise blood glucose levels similarly. Blood glucose management is not the reason to ax sugars and sweets, your health and weight are.

There are two important caveats to this advice:

1. The recommendations about the consumption of sugars and sweets for people with diabetes are the same as for the general public: Eat sugars and sweets in moderation.

2. Most people with pre-diabetes or type 2 diabetes need to lose weight and keep it off, as well as hit their blood glucose and blood lipid targets. Achieving these important goals doesn't leave much room for sugars and sweets, because they're chock full of calories, contain minimal nutrients, and may contain unhealthy fats.

With these caveats in mind, the ADA encourages you to fit sweets into your healthy eating plan on occasion, keeping in mind your weight, blood glucose, and blood lipid levels and goals.

The chart on pages 226–230 at the end of the chapter shows the serving size for sweets, along with information on calories, carbohydrate, total fat, saturated fat, and cholesterol content.

Sugars and the Nutrition Facts Label
Total Carbohydrate and Sugars

When you pick up a food and review the Nutrition Facts label, you may zero in on the sugars because you think they deserve your utmost attention; however, that's not true. Look at the Nutrition Facts for fat-free milk below, and you'll notice "Sugars" indented under the bold "Total Carbohydrate." The grams of sugars are accounted for within the grams of total carbohydrate. The grams of sugars in a food are a total of both the natural and the added sugars in one serving.

The term "Sugars," according to the FDA definition, includes all the one- and two-unit sugars. A one-unit sugar is glucose or fructose. A two-unit sugar is sucrose, made up of glucose and fructose, or lactose, made up of galactose and glucose. Two-unit sugars are common in some foods, such as fruit and milk. The label on the left shows that there are 11 grams of sugars and 12 grams of total carbohydrate in one serving of fat free milk. So, sugars account for most of the carbohydrate in the milk. Does milk have added sugar? No, the sugars are the natural milk sugars—lactose—found in dairy foods.

The Nutrition Facts label doesn't tell you whether the

FAT-FREE MILK

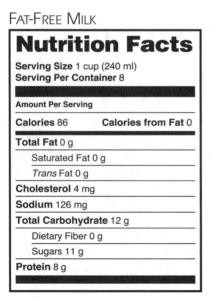

Nutrition Facts

Serving Size 1 cup (240 ml)
Serving Per Container 8

Amount Per Serving

Calories 86   Calories from Fat 0

Total Fat 0 g

   Saturated Fat 0 g

   Trans Fat 0 g

Cholesterol 4 mg

Sodium 126 mg

Total Carbohydrate 12 g

   Dietary Fiber 0 g

   Sugars 11 g

Protein 8 g

sugars are from natural or added sources. You can gain insight into the sources of sugars in a food from the reading the ingredients (ingredients are listed in descending order by weight used in the product).

Fructose, Honey, etc.

Are fructose, honey, agave nectar, and evaporated cane juice better

> ● QUICK TIP
>
> The key message from the Nutrition Facts label is to pay attention to the total carbohydrate count. Remember, all sources of carbohydrate, including natural or added sugars, raise your blood glucose.

than sugar? No. Fructose, honey, fruit juice concentrates, and other sweeteners raise blood glucose just like other sugars. One is no healthier than another. They have about the same number of calories and, other than fructose (this is not high fructose corn syrup, which contains about half fructose and half glucose), raise blood glucose at about the same speed. Fructose does raise blood glucose more slowly, but it might raise blood cholesterol if consumed in large amounts, which is not good.

Reduced-Calorie Sweeteners

There are two main groups of reduced-calorie sweeteners used in sugar-free foods today:

1. Sugar substitutes or no-calorie sweeteners (also called non-nutritive sweeteners)
2. Polyols, also called sugar alcohols.

Sugar Substitutes (No-Calorie Sweeteners)

Today there are five no-calorie sweeteners that have been approved through the FDA's food additive approval process and a newer group of stevia-based sweeteners, which have been approved through another FDA process called GRAS (Generally Recognized as Safe). All of these sweeteners have undergone lengthy safety research and reviews and have been shown to be safe for everyone including people with diabetes and pregnant women.

The no-calorie sweeteners approved as food additives are:
- acesulfame potassium (common brand name Sunette)
- aspartame (NutraSweet)
- neotame
- saccharin (Sweet 'n Low)
- sucralose (Splenda)

The main no-calorie sweeteners used today are aspartame and sucralose. They are found in many foods and beverages, including diet sodas, fruit drinks, syrups, yogurts, ice cream, jams, and other products. They are also available in packets or as granulated products to use like sugar for sweetening foods or for cooking and baking. The sweeteners contain almost no calories or carbohydrate, and they don't raise your blood glucose. They do contain a few calories contributed by carbohydrate-based bulking ingredients such as dextrose and maltodextrin.

> ● **Q U I C K   T I P**
>
> As long as you don't use more than 10 packets or teaspoons a day, you don't need to be concerned with the few calories and grams of carbohydrate from no-calorie sweeteners.

The no-calorie sweeteners approved as GRAS are similar forms of highly purified stevia called Rebaudioside A (Reb A or rebiana). (This is not the same product as the stevia sold as a dietary supplement.) The highly-purified form of stevia is extracted from the stevia plant which is native to Central and South America. There are now several highly purified based stevia sweeteners available a both a tabletop sweetener and available to manufacturers to use in foods and beverages. Several commercial names of these are: PureVia, Sun Crystals, Stevia in the Raw, and Truvia. The different tabletop sweeteners combine stevia with varied carbohydrate-based bulking ingredients, which contain a few calories from erythritol or cane sugar. They can be used in your eating plan similarly to other no-calorie sweeteners. You will note on the packaging and advertising that this group of sweeteners are referred to as natural; however, there is no official FDA definition of "natural." No research shows that stevia-based sweeteners offer you a health advantage over other no-calorie sweeteners. It is expected that other stevia-based sweeteners will make their way to the market.

Sugar substitutes can help you greatly lower the carbohydrates and calories you eat. Here is a comparison between a regularly sweetened fruit drink and a fruit drink sweetened with a no-calorie sweetener:

Type of Drink	Serving Size	Calories	Carbohydrate (g)	Sugars (g)
Regularly sweetened fruit drink	8 ounces	110	30	29
No-calorie fruit drink	8 ounces	10	2	0

Polyols (Sugar Alcohols)

Sugar alcohols are a group of ingredients commonly used in sugar-free foods. Interestingly, they're not sugar or alcohol. Rather, they are carbohydrate-based ingredients that contain, on average, half the calories of sugars (2 calories vs. 4 calories per gram). Polyols can replace sugar in foods such as candy, cookies, and ice creams.

Common names are: isomalt, sorbitol, lactitol, maltitol, mannitol, and xylitol. Note the common "ol" ending. Polyols contain about half the calories of sugar because they aren't completely digested. A downside of polyols is that in large amounts and in some people they can cause gas, cramps, and/or diarrhea. Some people, especially children, may be bothered by this side effect. Foods with certain amounts of polyols must contain an FDA-required statement on the label about this possible "laxative effect."

Replacing sugars with polyols in a food can cause a lower rise in blood glucose than with regularly sweetened foods; however, people don't tend to use these foods frequently enough to result in a significant lowering of calorie or carbohydrate intake or blood glucose. The calories and grams of carbohydrate per serving of sugar-free foods sweetened with polyols often are only minimally reduced. Here is a comparison of regular ice cream and ice cream sweetened with a sugar alcohol:

Type of Ice Cream	Serving Size	Calories	Total Fat (g)	Carbohydrate (g)	Sugars (g)	Sugar Alcohol (g)
Regular	1/2 cup	140	8	15	15	0
No-sugar-added, light	1/2 cup	100	5	15	4	3

Blends of Added Sugars and Reduced-Calorie Sweeteners

The availability of more polyols and no-calorie sweeteners has allowed food manufacturers to create a wider variety of sugar-free and lower-sugar foods. Some examples are calorie-free diet soda sweetened with one or a blend of no-calorie sweeteners, sugar-free ice cream sweetened with a no-calorie sweetener and one or more polyol, and blended sweeteners for baking that combine sugar and a no-calorie sweetener. Before you buy a product, read the ingredients to find out which sweeteners are used.

Sugar-Free Foods

If you choose to use foods with polyols and/or no-calorie sweeteners, read the ingredients, the Nutrition Facts label, and the chart on page 221 to figure out how to fit these foods into your healthy eating plan. Some of these foods can help you quench your sweet tooth without putting you over the top of your added sugars count.

So, how can you fit foods with polyols into your eating plan? If a food contains more than 5 grams of sugar alcohols, subtract half the grams of sugar alcohol from the carbohydrate grams to get the total carbohydrate grams to count in your eating plan.

How Sugar-Free Foods Fit into Your Eating Plan

If the Food Contains . . .	Count It as . . .
0–5 grams of total carbohydrate	a free food (limit to no more than 3 times a day)
6–10 grams of total carbohydrate	1/2 starch, fruit, or milk serving
11–20 grams of total carbohydrate	1 starch, fruit, or milk serving
21–25 grams of total carbohydrate	1 1/2 starch, fruit, or milk servings
26–35 grams of total carbohydrate	2 starch, fruit, or milk servings

Sugar-Free Hard Candy

Here's an example: This sugar-free hard candy contains 20 grams of sugar alcohols.

1/2 of the 20 grams of polyols = **10 grams**

Subtract that number from the grams of total carbohydrate:

28 grams of total carbohydrate – 10 grams =
18 grams of carbohydrate. That would be the equivalent of 1 starch, fruit, or milk serving.

Sugar-free Hard Candy (sweetened with maltitol and sorbitol)

Serving Size	10 pieces
Calories	80
Carbohydrate	36 g
Sugar Alcohols	31 g

The "Sugar-Free" Nutrition Claim Foods and beverages labeled "sugar-free" or alternatively "no sugar added" aren't necessarily carbohydrate or calorie free. The calorie count depends on which sweeteners (added polyols or sugar substitutes) have been used in the food as well as the other ingredients. Remember, according to the FDA's definition, "sugars" are defined as all one- and two-unit sugars, such as high fructose corn syrup, dextrose, or honey. The calorie-containing sweetening ingredients in some sugar-free foods, such as sorbitol and mannitol, aren't "sugars" by the FDA definition, but they still contain carbohydrate and calories. The sugar substitutes in some sugar-free foods don't contain calories or carbohydrate. Whether or not sugar-free foods cause a rise in blood glucose depends on the sweeteners and other ingredients in the food.

There is no doubt that many sugar-free foods—especially those sweetened with no-calorie sweeteners, such as diet carbonated and noncarbonated drinks, hot cocoa, yogurt, and syrups—can help satisfy your sweet tooth, reduce your waistline, lower your blood glucose, and perhaps improve your blood lipids. (That is as long as you consume them as part of an otherwise healthy lifestyle.) Explore a variety of sugar-free foods. Find a few that truly offer you a calorie savings and help you stay on track with your nutrition and diabetes goals.

Fitting in Sugars and Sweets

When you choose to eat sugary foods or sweets, substitute them for other carbohydrate in your eating plan or burn more calories. Consider these questions when you decide how many sugary foods and sweets to eat:

- Are my blood glucose and A1C on target or higher than desirable?
- Do I need to lose weight, so that I cannot afford a lot of calories as sugars and sweets?
- Are my blood fats—LDL, HDL, and triglycerides—in the target range?
- How much do I enjoy sugars and sweets, and how often do I feel I need to have a small serving to stay on track?
- Can I be more physically active after eating sugars and sweets to burn the extra calories and glucose?

Tips to Keep Added Sugars and Sweets to a Minimum

- Prioritize your personal diabetes goals. Which is most critical for you, keeping your blood glucose levels on target, losing weight, or lowering your blood lipids? Your priorities should dictate how you strike the balance with sugars and sweets.
- Choose a few favorite desserts and decide how often to eat them in light of your personal diabetes goals—maybe twice a week, just when dining out, or only at a special celebration.
- Note the calories, total fat, saturated fat, and cholesterol of the desserts you prefer. Then make your choices with these numbers and your diabetes goals in mind.
- Satisfy your sweet tooth with a small portion of your favorite sweet. Don't waste your calories on just so-so sweets.
- Split desserts when you eat out (at least in half).
- Take advantage of smaller portions when you can (kiddie or one scoop servings for ice cream).
- Use the Nutrition Facts on the food label to learn the grams of carbohydrate per serving. You need this information to swap a sweet food for other carbohydrate in your meal plan.
- Check the Nutrition Facts for the grams of sugars under total carbohydrate, and read the ingredients to try to decipher natural and added sugars.
- When you eat a sweet, check your blood glucose 1 to 2 hours afterward to see its effect. You might find that the same quantity of ice cream raises your blood glucose more slowly than frozen yogurt, which contains less fat and more carbohydrate. Let this information help you decide which sweets to eat, when to eat them, and how much to eat.
- Explore sugar-free options. With some foods, such as diet drinks and coffee sweeteners, it's a no-brainer and can save you a boatload of calories. Learn to cook and bake with a no-calorie sweetener. Find a few foods that truly save calories and satisfy your sweet tooth.

John's Story

John is an active high school senior who has had type 1 diabetes for 8 years. He plays several high school sports and is in the middle of basketball season on the varsity team. He takes rapid-acting insulin before each meal and long-acting insulin in the morning and at bedtime. He finds it easier to adjust his food and insulin with the flexibility of taking a shot of rapid-acting insulin before meals.

John is 6 feet 2 and weighs 182 pounds. Because of his high activity level he needs at least 3,000 calories a day. He actually has to work to keep his weight up. John has normal blood lipid levels and his blood glucose is generally on target.

When John recently met a dietitian for a review, John learned that the guidelines about sweets have changed since John developed diabetes. They discussed how John would work sweets into his eating plan and how to adjust his rapid-acting insulin to do so.

The dietitian asked John to name his favorite sweets. He listed peach cobbler, butter pecan ice cream, and chocolate chip cookies. She showed him how to substitute a reasonable portion of these sweets into his eating plan by adjusting his rapid-acting insulin at mealtime or when eating sweets as a snack based on the amount of carbohydrate in the sweets.

They decided it would make sense for John to eat a sweet at dinner on the days that he has basketball practice or a game in the afternoon. Other times, a sweet might fit in at lunch or as a snack before a sports practice. They decided that three or four times a week is a reasonable number of servings of sweets.

To see how sweets affect his diabetes, John will check his blood glucose about 1 to 2 hours after he eats sweets. He will determine his response to his favorite sweets and make adjustments in his rapid-acting insulin dosing if need be. John will also keep an eye on his blood lipid levels to observe any changes in the wrong directions.

Sharon's Story

Sharon is a 67-year-old retired school teacher. She was recently diagnosed with type 2 diabetes. She has about 25 pounds to lose, but her first goal is to lose 10 pounds. Besides high blood glucose levels and an A1C of 8.7%, she also has high triglycerides. Sharon has a sweet tooth; she is used to having at least one "sweet treat" every day. Since she met with a dietitian, she is trying to eat 1,200–1,400 calories a day, with no more than 35–45 grams of fat (about 30%).

Her dietitian suggested that Sharon fit in a sweet treat once or twice a week and that she eat them only when she has a meal away from home to help her limit the portions. She is keeping sweets out of her house because she believes she will eat them too often and in large quantities if they are there. Her choices are often a small serving of frozen yogurt, light ice cream, or splitting a dessert in a restaurant when she eats out.

Her dietitian suggested that she keep sugar-free hot cocoa mix, popsicles, and gingersnaps around to help satisfy her sweet tooth at other times.

Serving Sizes for Sugars and Sweets

Food	Serving Size	Calories	Carb (g)	Fat (g)	Saturated Fat (g)	Cholesterol (mg)
BEVERAGES, SODAS, AND ENERGY/SPORTS DRINKS						
Cranberry juice cocktail	1/2 cup	68	17.1	0.1	0.0	0
Energy drink	1 can (8.3 fl oz)	125	32.5	0.2	0.0	0
Fruit punch drink	1 cup (8 fl oz)	97	4.8	0.0	0.0	0
Hot chocolate (cocoa)	1 envelope (0.7 oz)	80	15.0	3.0	2.0	0
Hot chocolate (cocoa), sugar free	1 envelope (0.53 oz)	50	9.9	0.4	0.1	1
Hot cocoa mix, lite	1 envelope (.75 oz)	80	7.0	1.0	0.0	0
Lemonade, prepared	1 cup (8 fl oz)	112	28.7	0.0	0.0	0
Soft drink (soda), regular	1 can (12 fl oz)	147	37.6	0.0	0.0	0
Sports drink	1 cup	50	14.0	0.0	0.0	0
BROWNIES, CAKE, COOKIES, GELATIN, PIE, AND PUDDING						
Angel food cake, not frosted	1 slice (about 2 oz)	128	29.4	0.2	0.0	0
Brownie, small, unfrosted	1 brownie (1 1/4" sq, 7/8" high)	115	18.1	4.6	1.2	5
Cake, frosted	1 square (2")	175	29.2	6.4	2.0	18
Cake, unfrosted	1 square (2")	97	16.6	3.1	1.0	18

Food	Serving					
Cookies, chocolate chip	2 cookie, medium (2 1/4" dia)	156	18.7	9.1	2.6	10
Cookies, gingersnap, regular	3 cookies	87	16.1	2.1	0.5	0
Cookies, sandwich, cream filling	2 cookies, small	93	14.3	3.8	0.7	0
Cookies, sugar-free	3 cookies, small	141	20.4	6.9	1.8	0
Cookies, vanilla wafers	5 wafers	88	14.7	3.0	0.8	10
Cupcake, frosted, small	1 cupcake, small	174	29.2	6.1	1.3	8
Fruit cobbler	1/2 cup	84	19.2	0.0	0.0	0
Pie, fruit, 2 crust	1 slice (1/6th pie)	284	42.4	12.5	2.0	0
Pie, pumpkin or custard	1 slice (1/8th pie)	168	21.8	7.6	1.4	16
Pudding, regular (reduced-fat milk)	1/2 cup	141	25.9	2.4	1.4	10
Pudding, sugar-free, fat-free (fat-free milk)	1/2 cup	70	11.9	0.2	0.0	2
CANDY, SPREADS, SWEETS, SWEETENERS, SYRUPS, AND TOPPINGS						
Candy bar, chocolate or peanut type	2 bars, fun size (1/2 oz each)	151	19.8	7.5	2.6	2
Candy, hard	3 pieces	59	14.7	0.0	0.0	0
Chocolate kisses	5 kisses	105	12.2	6.1	3.7	3
Coffee creamer, dry, flavored	4 tsps	60	9.0	2.3	1.5	0

(continues)

Adapted from *Choose Your Foods: Exchange Lists for Diabetes* (American Dietetic Association and American Diabetes Association, 2008).

Serving Sizes for Sugars and Sweets (continued)

Food	Serving Size	Calories	Carb (g)	Fat (g)	Saturated Fat (g)	Cholesterol (mg)
Coffee creamer, liquid, flavored	2 tbsps	70	11.0	3.0	0.6	0
Fruit snacks (chewy rolls)	1 roll	78	17.7	1.5	0.0	0
Fruit spread, 100% fruit (jam, preserves)	1 1/2 tbsp	60	15.0	0.0	0.0	0
Honey, strained	1 tbsp	64	17.3	0.0	0.0	0
Jam or preserves, regular	1 tbsp	48	12.9	0.0	0.0	0
Jelly, regular	1 tbsp	52	13.4	0.0	0.0	0
Sugar, white, granulated	1 tbsp	48	12.5	0.0	0.0	0
Syrup, chocolate	2 tbsps	109	25.4	0.4	0.2	0
Syrup, pancake type, light	2 tbsps	50	13.0	0.0	0.0	0
Syrup, pancake type, regular	1 tbsp	50	13.2	0.0	0.0	0
CONDIMENTS AND SAUCES						
Barbecue sauce, bottled	3 tbsps	79	19.0	0.2	0.0	0
Cranberry sauce, canned, sugar added	1/4 cup	104	26.8	0.1	0.0	0
Gravy, canned or bottled	1/2 cup	53	6.4	0	0.3	1

Salad dressing, fat-free/low-fat, cream-based	3 tbsps	63	15.4	0.1	0.0	0
Sauce, sweet and sour	3 tbsps	67	16.1	0.0	0.0	0

DOUGHNUTS, MUFFINS, PASTRIES, AND SWEET BREADS

Banana nut bread	1 slice (1" thick)	178	30.5	5.4	2.2	34
Danish pastry, fruit type	1 pastry (4 1/4" dia)	263	33.9	13.1	3.5	81
Doughnut, cake-type, plain	1 medium	196	21.4	11.1	3.3	4
Doughnut, yeast type, glazed	1 doughnut (3 3/4" dia)	239	30.4	11.5	3.3	18
Muffin	0.25 large	103	12.9	5.0	2.0	16
Sweet roll	1 roll	264	36.1	11.6	2.2	47

FROZEN BARS, FROZEN DESSERTS, FROZEN YOGURT, AND ICE CREAM

Frozen pops, juice type	1 pop	27	6.5	0.1	0.0	0
Fruit juice bar, frozen, 100% juice	1 bar (3 oz)	75	18.6	0.1	0.0	0
Ice cream	1/2 cup	165	15.0	10.0	4.5	23
Ice cream, fat free	1/2 cup	90	22.0	0.0	0.0	0
Ice cream, light	1/2 cup	120	16.0	5.0	2.0	15
Ice cream, no sugar added	1/2 cup	115	14.5	5.5	2.3	10
Sherbet	1/2 cup	138	29.2	1.9	1.1	0

(continues)

Adapted from *Choose Your Foods: Exchange Lists for Diabetes* (American Dietetic Association and American Diabetes Association, 2008).

Serving Sizes for Sugars and Sweets *(continued)*

Food	Serving Size	Calories	Carb (g)	Fat (g)	Saturated Fat (g)	Cholesterol (mg)
Sorbet	1/2 cup	130	31.2	0.0	0.0	0
Yogurt, frozen, fat-free	1/3 cup	66	13.2	0.0	0.0	5
Yogurt, frozen, regular	1/2 cup	110	18.5	3.3	1.7	10
GRANOLA BARS, MEAL REPLACEMENT BARS/SHAKES, AND TRAIL MIX						
Granola bar	1 bar (1 oz)	134	18.3	5.6	1.0	0
Granola bar, chewy, low-fat	1 bar (1 oz)	109	21.9	2.0	0.5	0
Meal replacement bar, medium	1 bar (2 oz)	202	27.0	5.3	3.0	2
Meal replacement bar, small	1 bar (1 1/3 oz)	140	21.5	4.2	1.8	2
Meal replacement shake, reduced-calorie	1 can (10–11 oz)	220	38.0	3.0	0.5	5
Trail mix, candy and nut based	1 oz	137	12.7	9.0	1.7	1
Trail mix, fruit-based	1 oz	115	18.6	4.8	2.4	0

Adapted from *Choose Your Foods: Exchange Lists for Diabetes* (American Dietetic Association and American Diabetes Association, 2008).

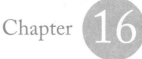

Chapter **16**

Beverages: Nonalcoholic

What You'll Learn:

- what's in the category of nonalcoholic beverages
- healthier and less-than-healthy beverages to choose
- the health hazards of beverages with added sugars
- the amount of added sugars in nonalcoholic beverages
- questions to ask yourself to get to know your current habits
- how easy it is to tank up on lots of calories from beverages
- tips to sip by

Nonalcoholic beverages don't constitute a food group, but many people today down more than 500 calories as they sip their favorite hot or cold beverages. You may not be conscious of the calories you are consuming, but they add up fast. Becoming aware of what's in your beverages and learning to choose healthier beverages can be a painless way to cut calories and lose weight, as well as control blood glucose.

Over the last two decades, the number of beverage choices has grown exponentially. Today, you can choose from regularly sweetened soda and diet soda to fruit drinks, flavored seltzers, bottles of fruit juice, sport drinks, hot or iced coffee with syrups and whipped cream, green and chai tea, and even sippable yogurt.

Unfortunately, many of these new categories of beverages are sweetened with sugars or syrups—namely, high fructose corn syrup. Many of them add loads of calories and grams of carbohydrate without adding anything nutritious. Thankfully, however, there are also more beverages sweetened with no-calorie sweeteners.

Here are some less-healthy beverages with added sugars and some healthier alternatives:

Less-Healthy Beverages with Added Sugars	Healthier Beverages with No Calories
Soda, regularly sweetened or sweetened with a combination of regular sweeteners and no-calorie sweetener	Water; mineral water, sparkling or still; diet soda; club soda; diet tonic water; seltzer, flavored with no sweetener
Fruit drinks, punches, ades	Fruit punch, with no-calorie sweetener
Sport drinks, regular	Sports drink, with no-calorie sweetener
Fruit juice made with 100% juice and fortified*	Fruit punch, with no-calorie sweetener; seltzer, flavored with no sweetener
Coffee, hot or iced, with syrup and whipped cream	Coffee sweetened with no-calorie sweetener
Tea with added sugars	Tea sweetened with no-calorie sweetener

*Though it is best to get your fruit as pieces of fresh, canned, frozen, or dried fruit, 100% fruit juice contains many nutrients. If you drink fruit juice, choose one that is fortified with calcium or other nutrients you need. Also measure the amounts you drink. A few ounces is not much.

Health Concerns Attributed to Beverages with Added Sugars

- The average person consumes about one third of their added sugars per day from regularly sweetened soda.
- People who drink regularly sweetened beverages are more likely to gain weight.
- People who eat and drink more added sugars tend to consume more calories, yet they don't get the nutrition they need. They eat insufficient amounts of foods that provide dietary fiber, vitamins, and minerals (fruits, vegetables, whole grains, etc.).
- Calories sipped as liquids may be more likely to cause weight gain than calories eaten as solid foods.

Nonalcoholic Beverages: How People Sip

Due in part to all these high-sugar beverages, the intake of added sugars has steadily risen over the last two decades. On average, people eat about 22 teaspoons of added sugars every day—over 355 calories. That's not hard to believe when you remember that a 20-ounce regularly sweetened soft drink contains about 15 teaspoons of added sugars (250 calories). In fact, regularly sweetened beverages contribute over 30% of the added sugar intake. There are also great nutrition and health concerns for children who consume high levels of added sugars. To learn more about sugars, see chapter 15.

> ● QUICK TIP
>
> Don't forget good old water—always the best beverage of choice. With zero calories, it's the best way to stay hydrated without any calories.

Get to Know Yourself

If you want to change your habits, you need to know what you drink now. Ask yourself these questions:

- What beverages do I drink day to day and in what quantities?
- How many calories do the beverages I drink add up to in a day?
- What changes am I willing to make in the beverages I choose to drink?

Nutrition Facts Tell the Truth

Don't be led astray with the word natural, the healthy pictures of fresh fruit on regularly sweetened drinks and drinkable yogurts, or the glowing advertisements about athletic performance on sports drinks. This is mostly hype. To find out what's really in the bottle or can, look to the Nutrition Facts label. Check out the serving size, calories, and carbohydrate. If the drink contains no calories or grams of carbohydrate, then it is probably not sweetened with added sugars. To know for sure, check the ingredients. High fructose corn syrup is the sweetener you find in most regularly sweetened bottled or canned drinks. You might also see the words corn sweetener, corn syrup, fruit juice concentrate, dextrose, glucose, or malt syrup.

Another food labeling law requires manufacturers to tell you the exact percentage of fruit juice used in a fruit beverage. Manufacturers can only use the term juice if the product is 100% fruit juice. A fruit "drink," like many of the products on the supermarket and convenience store shelves today, only has to contain 10% fruit juice. Some of them contain more, but most of these drinks are sweetened with added sugars.

It's Easy to Tank Up

Look how easy it is to tank up on a lot of calories and grams of carbohydrate just from one day of beverages.

Name of Drink	Amount	Calories	Carb (g)
Orange juice	12 ounces	164	38
Whole milk	8 ounces	150	12
Soda, regular	20-ounce bottle	258	66
Sport drink, regular	16-ounce bottle	112	28
Coffee frappe, blended coffee drink	16 ounces	260	52
Totals		944	196

See how changing your beverage choices can make a big dent in your calorie and carbohydrate totals.

Name of Drink	Amount	Calories	Carb (g)
Orange juice	8 ounces	110	25
Fat-free milk	8 ounces	90	12
Diet soda	20-ounce bottle	0	0
Sport drink, sweetened with no-calorie sweetener	16-ounce bottle	20	4
Cappuccino, sweetened with no-calories fat-free milk	16 ounces	100	14
Totals		320	55

In total, that's about 624 fewer calories and 141 fewer grams of carbohydrate. And it's simple and easy to do!

Healthier Ways to Quench Your Thirst

Instead of reaching for a beverage sweetened with added sugars, try these healthy tips:

- Quench your thirst with water. In most locales tap water is healthy and tasty.
- If you tire of water, choose club soda, seltzer, or sparkling water. To give water or these other drinks a new flavor at home or in restaurants, squeeze in a splash of lemon, lime, or orange.
- When you choose milk, opt for fat-free milk. If you just can't stand fat-free, use no more than 1% milk.
- When you choose juice, make sure it's 100% fruit juice and limit the amount you drink. If possible, buy the 100% juice fortified with calcium or Vitamin D.
- Stock your home with healthy drinks only—fat-free milk, fortified 100% juice, and water. Make these the options for meals and snacks for both kids and adults.
- If you choose a drinkable or squeeze yogurt, make sure it's sweetened with a no-calorie sweetener.
- If you drink soda, select a diet soda sweetened with one or more no-calorie sweeteners (sugar substitutes).
- Sweeten your coffee or tea with a no-calorie sweetener.
- If you order a specialty coffee or tea, order it made with fat-free milk. Sweeten it with a no-calorie sweetener.
- When you make iced tea, lemonade, or a dry-powdered fruit drink, like Kool-Aid or Crystal Light, sweeten it with a no-calorie sweetener rather than sugar or buy a ready made low-calorie drink.
- If you buy a sport drink, iced tea, or fruit drink, make it one sweetened with a no-calorie sweetener, such as Propel.
- When you eat in restaurants, opt for water, diet soda, 100% fruit juice, or low-fat milk.

Jerry's Story

Jerry just found out he has pre-diabetes. He is the youngest in his family, and three of his four siblings already have type 2 diabetes. He knew it was just a matter of time. Jerry is 45 years old, and he runs a lawn maintenance company. He used to do the physical labor, but now he finds himself behind a desk or riding around in his truck more than he used to.

Over the last 10 years, he has packed on 20 pounds at about two pounds per year. He was just told by his doctor that his blood pressure is a bit high, as are his triglycerides. Everything else seems normal. Jerry has young children, and he wants to be around when they get older. Both he and his wife need to shed some pounds.

Jerry was referred to a dietitian. He made an appointment and brought his wife along as the dietitian suggested. One question the dietitian asked Jerry was what nonalcoholic beverages he drinks. He said he starts his day with a couple cups of coffee with 2 teaspoons of sugar each and some half-and-half. Throughout the morning he sips on two more cups with cream and sugar. At lunch, he drinks a 20-ounce regularly sweetened soda, and throughout the afternoon he drinks a 20-ounce bottle of regularly sweetened sports drink. For dinner, he drinks regularly sweetened iced tea that they make up in bulk. He drinks no milk.

The dietitian made Jerry and his wife aware that he is drinking nearly 700 calories and 170 grams of carbohydrate a day in just beverages alone. They were astounded. She noted that an easy way for Jerry and his wife to trim some pounds is simply to change what he drinks. She suggested that he use a no-calorie sweetener in his coffee and iced tea. He said he would try the ones on the market to see what he likes best. She encouraged him to quench his thirst and stay hydrated with water, water, water, and when he wants a sweetened beverage, to choose one sweetened with a no-calorie sweetener. The dietitian also suggested that the whole family change to fat-free milk from 2% milk and that Jerry should drink at least two cups of fat-free milk a day. Jerry felt like these were some easy changes he and his family could make.

Chapter 17

Beverages: Alcoholic

What You'll Learn:

- the definition of a moderate amount of alcohol
- the definition of a serving of alcohol
- questions to ask yourself to get to know your current habits
- the upside and downside of drinking alcohol in general
- why, when, and how people with diabetes should or shouldn't drink alcohol
- what to be aware of if you have diabetes and choose to drink
- tips to sip alcohol by

> ● **Q U I C K   T I P**
>
> Alcohol can add a lot of calories (7 per gram) while offering essentially no nutrition.

Alcoholic beverages don't constitute a food group. You don't need alcohol to make up a well-balanced diet. There are some health benefits to drinking moderate amounts of alcohol; however, there are also some cautions to note. Some medicines you take and some diabetes-related or unrelated medical conditions may make drinking alcohol unwise.

Alcohol: How Much People Drink

People actually drink less alcohol today than they did a century ago. More than half of American adults drink alcohol today. General recommendations, as well as ADA recommendations, suggest you drink no more than a moderate amount of alcohol in a single day. A moderate amount is defined as one drink or serving of alcohol a day for women and two drinks a day for men. This amount should be consumed in a single day and not averaged over a few days at a time. Negative health effects have been noted with consumption of large amounts of alcohol at one sitting.

Alcohol Serving Sizes

A serving of alcohol is

- one 12-ounce regular beer,
- 5 ounces of wine (any type of wine other than dessert wine), or
- 1 1/2 ounces of 80-proof distilled spirits, such as gin or whiskey

Get to Know Yourself

If you want to change your habits, you need to know what you drink now. Ask yourself these questions:

- How many times a day or a week do I drink alcohol and how much?
- What types of alcohol do I drink?
- Do I mix alcohol with a mixer, such as juice, soda, or tonic water?
- How often would I like to drink alcohol?
- How many drinks are reasonable when I drink?

The Upside and Downside of Alcohol

Upside

From a health standpoint, some beneficial effects of a moderate amount of alcohol spread out over several days a week (rather than consuming large amounts of alcohol in one sitting) have been documented. In fact, light to moderate alcohol consumption has been linked to decreased risk of type 2 diabetes, heart disease, and stroke. The decrease in heart and blood vessel disease is thought to occur because alcohol can help increase HDL (good) cholesterol.

Alcohol has also been found to increase insulin sensitivity, which can help lower blood glucose. Light to moderate alcohol intake doesn't raise blood pressure; however, chronic excessive alcohol intake daily can raise blood pressure.

Interestingly, research shows that middle-aged and older people gain the most benefits from moderate alcohol intake. But don't start drinking alcohol because of these benefits if you don't currently drink. There are many other more powerful actions you can take to achieve your health goals, such as eating healthier foods, not smoking, and being physically active.

The upside of drinking a moderate amount of alcohol is the same for people with diabetes as it is in general. Because people with diabetes often have heart and blood vessel diseases, these benefits can be good news. Research shows that a moderate amount of alcohol, when consumed with food, has no quick effect on blood glucose or insulin levels.

Downside

Alcohol slows down physical and mental reaction time and can impair good judgment, including making healthier food choices. The effects of alcohol are dangerous for anyone behind the wheel of a car or for people near an intoxicated driver.

Excess alcohol consumption can cause or be a risk factor for liver disease (cirrhosis), high blood pressure, cancer in the organs of the gastrointestinal tract and other cancers, stroke, and motor vehicle accidents. Avoid alcohol if you are thinking of becoming pregnant, are currently pregnant or breastfeeding, have pancreatitis, have very high triglyceride levels, or have abused alcohol in the past.

> ● **QUICK TIP**
>
> Interestingly, women are more susceptible to the effects of alcohol than men. Some research points to a slight increased risk of breast cancer for women with even one drink a day or more.

From a nutrition standpoint, alcohol provides calories with essentially no nutrition. A couple of glasses of wine at dinner can quickly add up to 200 calories. If you are trying to eat 1,400 to 1,600 calories a day, 200 calories is nearly 15% of your calories. If you use up 200 calories as alcohol, you'll be hard pressed to get all the nutrients you need.

If you have diabetes, alcohol can cause blood glucose to go too low (hypoglycemia) and/or too high (hyperglycemia). The effect of alcohol on blood glucose depends on the amount of alcohol you drink at one time, whether or not you eat food when you drink, and if you take a blood glucose–lowering medication that can cause hypoglycemia.

Moderate amounts of alcohol can enhance the glucose-lowering effect of the insulin you take. Also, alcohol combined with some blood glucose–lowering oral medicines (see the list on page 244), as well as insulin, can cause blood glucose to get too low. The medications that can cause low blood glucose generally stimulate the pancreas to make or put out more insulin into the blood. Alcohol slows down the liver's ability to make new glucose to provide your body with energy. The result can be hypoglycemia, which will most likely affect you hours after you consume alcohol.

It is common to take more than one pill or one pill that contains a combination of two categories of these medicines. It is also common to take one or more pills and use an injectable medicine, such as insulin or an incretin mimetic. It may be that one medicine you take can cause hypoglycemia and another is unlikely to. Learn the actions of your medicines from your health care providers and your risks for low blood glucose episodes.

This is not a complete list of all blood glucose–lowering medicines approved by the FDA. Be aware that new blood glucose–lowering medications may be approved by the FDA for use from time to time. People who don't take insulin or one of these medicines which may cause low blood glucose have a much lower risk of hypoglycemia from alcohol.

Alcohol can also cause blood glucose to rise. Some alcoholic beverages, such as beer and wine, contain carbohydrate, as do mixers, such as orange juice or regular soda. Alcohol consumption can make some diabetes complications worse, such as diabetic neuropathy (nerve damage). Alcohol is toxic to nerves and can increase the pain, burning, tingling, numbness, and other symptoms of nerve damage. Heavy alcohol use can worsen diabetic eye disease, high blood pressure, and very high triglyceride levels.

Fitting Alcohol into Your Eating Plan

Current guidelines from the ADA suggest that you can factor alcoholic beverages into your eating plan in addition to the calories from foods and nonalcoholic beverages. Be aware that cutting calories to make room for the calories from alcohol can increase the risks of hypoglycemia in people on some medications (see page 244). If you are striving to lose weight, keep in mind that the calories from alcohol can add up quickly and add no nutrition.

Blood Glucose–lowering Medicines which May Cause Hypoglycemia

Pills you take by mouth		
Category Name	**Generic Names**	**Brand Names**
Sulfonylureas	glimepiride, glipizide, glyburide	Amaryl, Glucotrol, Glucatrol XL, Diabeta, Micronase
Meglitinides	repaglinide	Prandin
D-phenylalanine	nateglinide	Starlix
Insulins		
Insulin		all types

Blood Glucose–lowering Medicines Unlikely to Cause Hypoglycemia

Pills you take by mouth		
Biquanides	metformin	Glucophage, Glucophage XR, Glumetza, Fortamet, Riomet (liquid)
Glitazones (TZDs)	pioglitazone, rosiglitazone	Actos, Avandia
Alpha-glucosidase inhibitor	acarbose, miglitol	Precose, Glyset
DPP-4 inhibitors	sitagliptin saxagliptin	Januvia Onglyza
Bile sequestering agent (removes glucose and LDL-cholesterol from the body)	coles(s)evatam HCL	Welchol
Dopamine agonist	bromocriptine mesylate	Cycloset
Injectable medicines		
Incretin mimetics (work like gut hormones called incretins)	Exenatide	Byetta
Amylin analog (works like pancreas hormone amylin)	Pramlintide	Symlin (most often used with insulin, insulin doses usually need to be cut to prevent lows)

Which Alcoholic Drink Is Best?

Should you drink red wine or white wine, bourbon or whiskey, or regular beer or light beer? Research shows that any type of alcohol can have beneficial effects on the heart and blood vessels. It is best to drink as few calories and grams of carbohydrate as you can, so a shot of distilled spirits is better than a mixed drink with juice and grenadine syrup or one with regular soda. For mixers, stick with club soda, sparkling mineral water, diet tonic water, water, diet soda, tomato or V8 juice, Bloody Mary mix, or coffee (for a hot drink).

Alcohol Adds Flavor, Not Fat

A bit of wine, sherry, or liqueur can enhance the taste of foods and adds just a few calories. Alcohol is a wonderful low-fat cooking ingredient. You might stock red and white cooking wine, sherry, and liqueurs (clear ones, not creamy) in your pantry. Here are a few culinary ideas with alcohol:

- add sherry to a marinade for chicken or meat
- pour red cooking wine in a tomato sauce
- use white cooking wine in a poaching liquid
- add orange liqueur to a fruit salad
- dress up coffee with a spot of hazelnut liqueur
- drizzle a tablespoon of raspberry liqueur on frozen yogurt
- poach fruit in red wine.

Tips to Sip By

- Don't drink when your blood glucose is too low.
- If you take insulin or other diabetes medications that can cause low blood glucose (see chart, page 244), have a snack or meal with the alcohol if your blood glucose is too low when you start to drink.
- Check your blood glucose levels more often when you drink alcohol. These checks will help you learn more about the effect of alcohol on your body.
- Check your blood glucose before you drive a vehicle after you have had a drink to make sure your blood glucose is in a safe range. Do not drive if you believe you've had too much to drink and/or you are at risk of becoming hypoglycemic.
- The symptoms of intoxication and hypoglycemia can be similar. You don't want people to confuse these two, because they might not provide you with the proper treatment. Make sure you drink safely and wear a medical ID that says you have diabetes.
- Sip a drink slowly to make it last.
- Make a glass of wine last longer by making it a "spritzer." Mix the wine with sparkling water or club soda or diet ginger ale.
- Choose light beer over regular beer if you like it and want to save a few calories.
- Have a no-calorie beverage, like water, club soda, or diet soda, on the side to quench your thirst.

Jack's Story

Jack, age 47, has had type 2 diabetes for 3 years. He is trying to eat between 1,900 and 2,300 calories a day and to fit in a 1-mile walk three times a week. He takes a diabetes pill in the sulfonylurea category twice a day.

With this plan, Jack has shed 12 pounds over the last 15 months, and his blood glucose levels have improved. His A1C decreased from a high of 8.6% to 7.3%.

Jack travels a lot for work and finds himself at business dinners three nights a week. He usually has a cocktail of rum and diet cola on the rocks, wine with dinner, and, on occasion, an after-dinner liqueur. On the weekend, he might drink a few beers or several glasses of wine at a restaurant or while watching TV. See how fast the calories add up from one of Jack's business dinners:

Cocktail: 1 rum and diet cola (1 1/2 oz rum) = 96 calories
Wine: 1 glass white wine (5 oz) = 98 calories
After-dinner liqueur: Kahlua (1 1/2 oz) = 175 calories

These three drinks add up to almost 370 calories just from alcohol. That's about 20% of Jack's calories for the day.

Jack recognizes that the alcohol is not helping him lose weight. What he didn't know is that the diabetes medication he takes, glyburide, can cause his blood glucose to go too low. When he drinks, he increases his risk of hypoglycemia further. He now realizes he experienced this recently the morning after a light business dinner that included several alcoholic drinks. He became hypoglycemic in the early morning hours.

He knows it's time to start to decrease the amount of alcohol he drinks. Through the process of setting goals, Jack agrees to drink only light beer and to stop at two beers when he drinks beer. When he is on business trips, he'll drink either a cocktail or a glass of wine with dinner and skip the after-dinner liqueur. When he is out to dinner on the weekend, he will have no more than two glasses of wine.

To prevent hypoglycemia, he will check his blood glucose before bed after drinking in the evening. He will eat a snack if his blood glucose level is below 90 mg/dl before he goes to sleep.

Chapter 18

Combination, Convenience, and Free Foods

What You'll Learn:

- what are combination foods
- what are convenience foods
- how to fit combination and convenience foods into your healthy eating plan
- what are free foods
- the serving sizes and nutrition numbers for combination, convenience, and free foods

249

Combination Foods Defined

You have read a lot in section 2 about foods that fit nicely into different food groups. The way these foods divide into food groups makes perfect sense—apples in the fruit group, barley in the starch group, and pork chops in the meat group; however, most people also regularly enjoy combination foods or dishes—bean burritos, beef stew, shepherd's pie, or minestrone soup. The ingredients in bean burritos, for example, come from several food groups. Beans and tortillas are in the starch group, cheese is in the meat group, and lettuce, onion, and tomato are all in the vegetable group.

Convenience Foods Defined

Convenience foods are the packaged foods you buy in the supermarket or convenience store that are close to being ready-to-eat. Frozen pizza, a box of macaroni and cheese, and a lean frozen entrée are all convenience foods. To say that there's been an increase in the use of convenience foods in recent decades is an understatement. Today, people who prepare meals at home often do more "assembling" using convenience foods, than cooking from scratch.

A benefit of convenience foods is that they have Nutrition Facts labels and ingredients on the packaging that help you know what you're eating. This can be scary as well! This information is not often readily available, however, for some convenience foods, such as potato salad from the supermarket deli counter. The biggest nutritional downfall of many convenience foods, which are generally processed, is their high sodium content.

Later in this chapter, you'll find tips to help you make healthier convenience food choices. You can read chapter 22 to learn how to fit restaurant foods into your eating plan and access restaurant nutrition information.

Whether you make combination dishes from scratch, or purchase ready-to-eat-or-heat convenience foods, you'll need to figure out—or guesstimate—what's in them to determine how many servings the food contains from each food group.

Fitting in Foods When You Have a Recipe

Whether you choose to make a favorite old recipe or try a new one, you can learn how to fit a serving of these recipes (or convenience foods) into your healthy eating plan by following these steps:

1. Write down the amount of each ingredient used in the recipe. (There are websites that provide tools for you to do this quicker and easier.)

2. Find the grams of carbohydrate, protein, and fat in the amount of each ingredient. Use an online nutrient database resource such as ADA's My Food Advisor www.diabetes.org/food-nutrition-lifestyle/nutrition/my-food-advisor.jsp, or the USDA's searchable food database www.ars.usda.gov/main/site_main.htm?modecode=12-35-45, or use a book filled with the nutrient counts of foods, such as *The Ultimate Calories, Carb, and Fat Gram Counter*, ADA, 2006. Add up the total grams of carbohydrate, protein, and fat from all ingredients in the whole recipe.

3. Divide the total grams of carbohydrate, protein, and fat by the number of portions you will serve from the recipe.

Don't waste your effort. If you believe you'll prepare this recipe again and again, write down the nutrition information per servings on the recipe. Then you'll have it forever.

Here's an example using a recipe for Vegetarian Mexican Chili (next page).

Now think about the food groups represented in this recipe. You've got onions, peppers, and tomatoes from the vegetable group and beans and bulgur from the starch group. Spices and seasonings like garlic, chili powder, and cumin have essentially no calories, so they are free foods.

You know from the chapters on starches and vegetables that one starch serving has 15 grams of carbohydrate and 3 grams of protein. In this recipe, you have about three starch servings from the beans and bulgur. A vegetable serving contains 5 grams of carbohydrate and 2 grams of protein. The onions, peppers, and tomatoes in this recipe provide about two vegetable servings. Subtract these amounts from the amounts in one portion of the recipe as follows. Note that there

Vegetarian Mexican Chili

Ingredients	Amount	Carb (g)	Protein (g)	Fat (g)
Chopped onions	1 cup	16	2	0
Chopped red pepper	3/4 cup	7	1	0
Chopped green pepper	3/4 cup	5	1	0
Minced garlic	2 tsp	2	0	0
Kidney beans	2 (16-oz) cans	160	54	4
Stewed tomatoes	2 (14 1/2-oz) cans	55	8	2
Tomato paste	1 (6-oz) can	32	7	1
Bulgur, dry	2/3 cup	70	11	1
Chili powder	1 1/2 Tbsp	0	0	0
Cumin, ground	1 tsp	0	0	0
Totals for whole recipe		347	84	8
Totals for 1 portion (1/6 of recipe)		58	14	1

are a few grams of carbohydrate, protein, and fat remaining, but this is close enough. So, one portion of this Vegetarian Mexican Chili contains 3 starches and 2 vegetables—a mighty healthy dish.

Help from Diabetes and Healthy Eating Cookbooks and Online Recipe Sites

You'll find that many cookbooks or websites aimed at people with diabetes or people who want to eat healthier, provide you with essential

	Carb (g)	Protein (g)	Fat (g)
Totals for 1 portion (6 portions per recipe)	58	14	1
3 starch servings	– 45	– 9	0
after subtraction	13	5	1
2 vegetable servings	– 10	– 4	0
Remainder	3	1	1

nutrition information, such as the carbohydrate, protein, and fat content per serving. This information and the ingredient list can help you determine the number of servings from each food group.

Consider the example of a recipe for Chicken Paprikash from an ADA cookbook. The nutrition content for one serving is listed below. Next, we read the ingredients to see that it contains oil, chicken, onions, green pepper, frozen green beans, and fat-free sour cream. The recipe also includes many herbs and spices, such as parsley, bay leaf, garlic, and lemon juice. These are free foods. Use the ingredient list to see the food groups that are represented, and then use the same process as in the example with Vegetarian Mexican Chili. You may get extra help from some diabetes cookbooks that also provide you with the so-called diabetes exchanges for the recipes. All of the ADA cookbooks provide this information. You can figure that the diabetes exchanges are equivalent to the servings discussed in this book. For example, the exchanges for this Chicken Paprikash recipe are 2 vegetables and 3 lean meat.

	Carb (g)	Protein (g)	Fat (g)
Totals for 1 portion (7 portions per recipe)	17	25	7
3 vegetable servings	− 15	− 6	0
after subtraction	2	19	7
3 meat servings (lean)	0	21	9
Remainder	2	− 2	− 2

Fitting in Foods with a Food Label in Hand

You can use this same process to fit combination, convenience, or prepared foods into your eating plan. Perhaps you want to eat a frozen cheese pizza. From the Nutrition Facts label, get the grams of carbohydrate, protein, and fat. This information is per serving. From the ingredients list, learn which ingredients contribute these nutrients. Use this information and the process above to figure out the servings from the different food groups.

Nutrition Facts

Serving Size 1/6 pizza
Serving Per Container 6

Amount Per Serving

Calories 290   **Calories from Fat** 81

Total Fat 9 g
    Saturated Fat 4.5 g
    Trans Fat 0 g
Cholesterol 25 mg
Sodium 700 mg
Total Carbohydrate 42 g
    Dietary Fiber 2 g
    Sugars 5 g
Protein 11 g

Putting Together Meals with Convenience Foods

Ingredients: wheat flour, corn meal, dextrose, whole milk mozzarella cheese, tomato paste, asiago cheese, romano cheese. (Note: This is a partial list of ingredients; the others do not contribute calories or nutrients.)

If you use some of the healthier convenience foods available today, you can quickly put together a nutritious meal. You might combine a frozen pizza with a salad that you make at home or one you buy and then add an apple for dessert. You may opt for a frozen entrée that is healthy and combine it with a serving of leftover broccoli, a slice of whole-wheat bread, and glass of fat-free milk. There are many convenience foods to choose from. The following examples show you how you can use them to your advantage to put together healthy meals.

Sample Meal Plan with Convenience Foods

BREAKFAST: Frozen Waffles

2 frozen whole-grain waffles	2 starches
1 1/4 cups sliced strawberries	1 fruit
1 cup fat-free milk	1 milk

LUNCH: Frozen Pizza

2 slices pizza topped with red peppers, tomatoes, and mushrooms	3 starches 2 oz meat 2 vegetables
1 cup fat-free, sugar-free strawberry yogurt	1 milk
1 small banana sliced into yogurt	1 fruit

DINNER: Frozen Entrée

Chicken Oriental Stir-Fry	2 starches 1 vegetable 3 oz meat
1 small whole-wheat dinner roll	1 starch
Salad with lettuce, cucumbers, carrots, and sliced tomato	1 vegetable
1 tsp extra-virgin olive oil	1 fat
2 Tbsp balsamic vinegar	free food
1 cup fat-free milk	1 milk

Choosing Healthier Convenience Foods

Convenience foods are not necessarily as healthy as the same item made in your home. Some packaged and frozen foods are higher in salt and sodium and contain additives and preservatives. Others, like fresh fruits and vegetables, are just as healthy but offer the convenience of being washed, cut up, and/or ready to eat. Some packaged convenience foods may contain more fat, and especially the unhealthy trans fat, because they contain partially hydrogenated fat to keep them fresh in the supermarket. Does that mean you should not eat them?

Clearly, it would be best to make all your food from scratch, but most people can't or aren't willing to do this. Do try to use as few convenience foods as you can and select healthier convenience foods when you do buy them. For example, choose lower-sodium options, such as soup, broth, or canned vegetables. Choose frozen vegetables that don't have special sauces or seasonings. Add the herbs and spices yourself. Keep in mind that processed foods contribute about three quarters of the sodium we eat.

The chart at the end of this chapter provides the serving sizes for some popular convenience combination foods, along with their calorie, carbohydrate, protein, fat, saturated fat, and sodium content.

Free Foods

Free foods, as defined by the ADA, contain less than 20 calories or less than 5 grams of carbohydrate per serving. You'll find the list of free foods on pages 259–267 at the end of this chapter, along with serving size (if one is indicated), calories, carbohydrate, and sodium. Free foods with a serving size listed should be limited to three servings a day. Spread them out during the day. If you eat all three servings at one time, it could raise your blood glucose level. Foods listed without a serving size can be eaten whenever you want in whatever quantity (within reason) you want.

Sandy's Story

Sandy is 25 years old. She is single, and she has had type 1 diabetes for 8 years. She recently started her first job after finishing law school. She is adjusting to her new life as a hard-working attorney in a busy office. Sandy tries to stay on track with her diabetes. For breakfast, she eats a quick bowl of cereal with fruit, or she pops a whole-grain English muffin into the toaster and grabs a banana to eat on the way. She takes lunch from home—a sandwich, a piece of fruit, and a handful of pretzels. On the days that she goes out with colleagues or clients, she ends up overeating.

By the time she gets home at night, she is too tired and hungry to spend time cooking. She finds that the healthier convenience meals are satisfying and quick. She learned how to fit these meals into her eating plan. In general, they are 2 to 3 ounces of cooked meat, one starch, and one vegetable.

Her eating plan for dinner calls for 3 ounces of meat, two starches, two vegetables, one fruit, and one milk. Sandy knows that along with the frozen entrée, she needs to add a whole-wheat roll or crackers for another starch and a salad, sliced tomato, or handful of baby carrots for another vegetable. She adds a cup of fat-free milk and has a piece of fruit soon after dinner. Other evenings, Sandy grabs a quick meal out with friends or gets a takeout meal at a pizza or rotisserie-chicken shop.

Ray's Story

Ray is 72 years old and has been a widower for about a year. He has had type 2 diabetes for 3 years and takes two blood glucose–lowering pills before breakfast and dinner. Ray's wife did all the cooking, so he stocks a few frozen meals and bags of frozen vegetables in the freezer and keeps some canned goods on the shelf. Otherwise, he eats at nearby cafeterias.

Recently, Ray met with the registered dietitian he saw after he was first diagnosed with diabetes. His doctor asked him to go back because he has gained 8 pounds since his wife died and his blood glucose is climbing. The RD pointed out that Ray chooses some high-fat convenience foods. He buys the regular type of frozen meals and chooses chicken pot pie, meat loaf with gravy and potatoes, and lasagna. For vegetables, he chooses spinach soufflé, peas and onions in butter sauce, and broccoli in cheese sauce.

The RD suggested that Ray purchase products that are lower in fat, calories, and sodium and that come in smaller portions. She said that it is better to buy vegetables without cream, cheese, or butter sauce. If Ray wants to put a bit of a healthier margarine or spread on the vegetables after they are cooked, that is fine. However, a squeeze of lemon or lime juice, which is a free food, is even better.

In the cafeteria, Ray should order an entrée, one starch, two vegetables, and a salad with dressing on the side. She encouraged him to think about how his healthier plates should look. Some of the healthier entrées that Ray could order are meatloaf with tomato sauce, roast beef, roasted chicken, or boiled fish. The RD suggested that Ray ask for a take-home container when he orders his meal to avoid overeating. When he first sits down, he can put half the entrée in container to save for another meal. Then he can enjoy a reasonable amount of meat, starches, and vegetables. She encouraged him to watch out for the fats in fried foods, butter, sour cream, and creamy sauces on vegetables.

They discussed how many servings of foods from the different food groups Ray should eat each day and how some of his food selections fit in. She emphasized that 2 to 3 ounces of cooked meat equals one serving and that Ray's cafeteria choices are closer to 6 to 8 ounces—perfect for splitting into two portions.

Serving Sizes for Combination, Convenience, and Free Foods

Food	Serving Size	Calories	Carb (g)	Protein (g)	Fat (g)	Saturated Fat (g)	Sodium (mg)
COMBINATION FOODS: ENTREES							
Chili with beans	1 cup	336	28.0	19.4	16.2	7.4	1152
Lasagna with meat and sauce	1 cup	293	27.9	19.7	11.4	5.0	776
Macaroni and cheese	1 cup	283	35.4	10.8	11.0	6.2	1343
Spaghetti, sauce, meatballs	1 cup	273	28.3	10.6	13.0	5.0	1035
Stew, meat and vegetables	1 cup	160	17.0	12.5	5.2	2.2	990
Tuna noodle casserole	1 cup	295	32.3	21.3	8.4	2.3	448
Tuna or chicken salad	1/2 cup	182	7.0	15.3	10.3	1.7	328
COMBINATION FOODS: FROZEN ENTREES/MEALS							
Burrito (beef and bean)	1 burrito	350	45.0	12.5	13.4	5.0	560
Dinner-type meal, frozen	1 meal (16 oz)	513	54.0	26.8	20.9	6.8	1403
Entree or meal (<340 calories)	1 container (~9.5 oz)	299	40.4	18.3	6.7	2.2	535
Pizza, cheese, thin crust, frozen	1 1/4 th of 12"	291	33.0	13.5	12.5	6.0	565

(continues)

Adapted from *Choose Your Foods: Exchange Lists for Diabetes* (American Dietetic Association and American Diabetes Association, 2008).

Serving Sizes for Combination, Convenience, and Free Foods *(continued)*

Food	Serving Size	Calories	Carb (g)	Protein (g)	Fat (g)	Saturated Fat (g)	Sodium (mg)
Pizza, meat topping, thin crust, frozen	1 1/4 th of 12"	365	34.0	16.0	18.5	8.0	816
Pocket sandwich	1 sandwich	310	46.5	11.5	9.5	5.3	725
Pot pie, double crust	1 pie (7 oz)	390	39.3	9.7	21.3	6.7	778
COMBINATION FOODS: SALADS (DELI-STYLE)							
Coleslaw, deli style	1/2 cup	130	16.0	1.0	7.0	1.0	160
Macaroni or pasta salad, deli style	1/2 cup	280	28.0	4.0	14.0	2.0	430
Potato salad, mustard type, deli-style	1/2 cup	180	25.0	2.0	6.0	1.0	690
COMBINATION FOODS: SOUPS							
Chowder, made with milk	1 cup	190	19.0	6.5	9.8	2.5	865
Miso soup	1 cup	84	8.0	6.0	3.4	0.6	989
Oriental noodle soup (Ramen type)	1 cup	240	30.0	6.0	10.5	6.0	1031
Rice soup (congee)	1 cup	72	13.5	1.7	1.4	0.4	487

Soup, bean	1 cup	116	19.8	5.6	1.5	0.0	1198
Soup, chicken noodle, made with water	1 cup	75	9.4	4.0	2.5	1.0	1106
Soup, cream of celery, made with water	1 cup	90	8.8	1.7	5.6	1.0	949
Soup, cream of mushroom, made with water	1 cup	129	9.3	2.3	9.0	2.0	881
Soup, instant, 6 oz, prepared	1 envelope	65	11.1	1.9	1.6	0.5	561
Soup, instant, beans or lentils, prepared	1 container (2 oz)	215	39.4	12.2	1.5	0.0	523
Soup, split pea, made with water	1 cup	190	28.0	10.4	4.4	2.0	1012
Soup, tomato, made with water	1 cup	85	16.6	2.0	1.9	0.0	695
Soup, vegetable beef, made with water	1 cup	78	10.2	5.6	1.9	1.0	791

Adapted from *Choose Your Foods: Exchange Lists for Diabetes* (American Dietetic Association and American Diabetes Association, 2008).

Serving Sizes for Combination, Convenience, and Free Foods (continued)

Food	Serving Size	Calories	Carb (mg)	Sodium (mg)
FREE FOODS: LOW CARBOHYDRATE FOODS				
Arugula	1 cup	5	0.7	5
Beans, green, fresh, cooked	1/4 cup	11	2.4	0
Cabbage, green, fresh, raw	1/2 cup	8	2.0	6
Candy, hard, small size	1 piece, small	12	2.9	2
Candy, hard, sugar-free	1 candy	20	4.7	0
Carrots, fresh cooked	1/4 cup	18	4.1	25
Cauliflower, fresh cooked	1/4 cup	7	1.2	5
Chewing gum, regular	1 stick	7	2.0	0
Chicory greens, fresh, raw	1 cup	7	1.4	13
Cranberries, fresh, raw	1/2 cup	22	5.8	1
Cucumber, with peel	1/2 cup	8	1.9	1
Endive or escarole	1 cup	9	1.7	11
Gelatin dessert, sugar-free, all flavors	1/2 cup	8	0.1	56
Gelatin, unflavored	1 envelope	23	0.0	14
Jelly or preserves, low or reduced sugar	2 tsps	16	4.0	0
Lettuce, iceburg	1 cup	7	1.2	5

Food	Serving			
Radicchio	1/2 cup	5	0.9	4
Rhubarb, cooked (sweetened with sugar subst)	1/2 cup	25	5.4	5
Romaine, raw	1 cup	8	1.5	4
Spinach, fresh, raw	1 cup	7	1.1	24
Sugar substitute (Equal)	1 pkt	4	0.9	0
Sugar substitute, (Sugar Twin spoonable)	1 tsp	1	0.4	1
Sugar substitute (Splenda)	1 pkt	4	1.0	0
Syrup, sugar-free	2 tbsps	9	2.3	27
Watercress, fresh	1 cup	4	0.4	14
FREE FOODS: MODIFIED FAT FOODS WITH CARBOHYDRATE				
Cream cheese, fat-free	1 tbsp (1/2 oz)	17	1.2	116
Creamer, nondairy, liquid	1 tbsp	20	1.7	12
Creamer, nondairy, powder, regular	2 tsps	22	2.2	7
Margarine spread, fat-free	1 tbsp	6	0.6	81
Margarine, reduced-fat	1 tsp	16	0.0	29
Margarine-like spread, tub, light or reduced fat	1 tsp	16	0.0	29
Mayonnaise, fat-free	1 tbsp	11	2.3	120
Mayonnaise, reduced-fat	1 tsp	16	0.4	43

(continues)

Adapted from Choose Your Foods: Exchange Lists for Diabetes (American Dietetic Association and American Diabetes Association, 2008).

Serving Sizes for Combination, Convenience, and Free Foods (continued)

Food	Serving Size	Calories	Carb (mg)	Sodium (mg)
Mayonnaise-style salad dressing, fat-free	1 tbsp	13	2.5	126
Mayonnaise-style salad dressing, reduced fat	1 tsp	12	0.8	44
Salad dressing, fat-free	1 tbsp	20	4.5	145
Salad dressing, Italian, fat-free	2 tbsps	15	3.2	310
Salad dressing, low-fat	1 tbsp	19	2.5	176
Sour cream, fat-free	1 tbsp	11	0.5	8
Sour cream, reduced-fat	1 tbsp	22	1.1	13
Whipped topping, fat-free (Cool Whip)	2 tbsps	15	3.0	5
Whipped topping, lite (Cool Whip)	2 tbsps	20	3.0	0
Whipped topping, regular (Cool Whip)	1 tbsp	12	1.0	0
FREE FOODS: CONDIMENTS				
Barbecue sauce	2 tsps	17	4.2	130
Catsup (ketchup), tomato	1 tbsp	16	4.1	178
Cheese, parmesan, freshly grated	1 tbsp	25	0.2	45
Chili sauce, tomato-type, sweet	2 tsps	11	2.5	134
Honey mustard	1 tbsp	14	2.8	85

Horseradish	1 tbsp	7	1.7	47
Lemon juice	1 tbsp	3	1.0	3
Miso, soybean paste, fermented	1 1/2 tsps	17	2.3	319
Mustard, prepared	1 tsp	3	0.4	56
Pickles, dill	1 1/2 medium (3 3/4")	18	4.0	1250
Pickles, sweet, bread and butter	2 slices	16	4.5	131
Pickles, sweet, gherkin	3/4 oz	25	6.8	200
Relish, sweet pickle	1 tbsp	20	5.3	122
Salsa	1/4 cup	17	4.1	388
Soy sauce	1 tbsp	8	1.2	902
Soy sauce, light	1 tbsp	12	1.3	573
Sweet and sour sauce	2 tsps	15	3.6	51
Taco sauce	1 tbsp	10	2.0	120
Vinegar	1 tbsp	1	0.6	0
Yogurt, plain, nonfat milk	2 tbsps	17	2.4	23
FREE FOODS: FREE SNACKS				
Blueberries, fresh, free food size	1/4 cup	21	5.3	0
Carrots, baby, raw, free food size	5 baby carrots	12	2.8	20

(continues)

Adapted from *Choose Your Foods: Exchange Lists for Diabetes* (American Dietetic Association and American Diabetes Association, 2008).

Serving Sizes for Combination, Convenience, and Free Foods (continued)

Food	Serving Size	Calories	Carb (mg)	Sodium (mg)
Celery, fresh, raw, free food size	5 sticks (5" long)	12	2.5	68
Cheese, fat-free, free food size	1/2 oz	20	1.3	182
Cream pop, frozen, sugar-free	1 pop	20	4.8	2
Goldfish-style crackers, free snack size	10 goldfish crackers	30	3.8	50
Lean meat, cooked, free food size	1/2 oz	23	0.0	10
Popcorn, light, free food size	1 cup	22	4.7	52
Saltine-type crackers, free food size	2 crackers	26	4.3	64
Vanilla wafers, free food size	1 wafer	18	2.9	14
FREE FOODS: DRINKS/MIXES				
Bouillon, granules or cubes, beef or chicken	1 tsp	5	0.8	900
Bouillon, sodium free, instant powder	1 tsp	10	2.0	0
Broth, chicken, 99% fat free	1 cup	17	0.9	983
Broth, chicken, low sodium, canned	1 cup	32	1.6	113
Carbonated (mineral) water	1 cup	0	0.0	2
Club soda, regular	1 can (12 oz)	0	0.0	75

Food	Serving Size			
Cocoa, powder, unsweetened	1 tbsp	12	2.9	1
Coffee, brewed	1 cup	5	1.1	5
Diet soft drinks, sugar-free	1 can (12 oz)	4	0.3	35
Drink mix, sugar free lemonade	1/8 envelope	5	1.4	3
Tea, brewed	1 cup	3	0.5	7
Tonic water, sugar free	1 cup	0	0.0	35
Water, bottled, flavored, carbohydrate free	1 cup	0	0.0	7
Water, drinking (tap)	1 cup (8 fl oz)	0	0.0	9
FREE FOODS: SEASONINGS				
Basil, dried	1 tsp, leaves	2	0.4	0
Basil, fresh, leaves	1 tbsp	1	0.1	0
Cooking Spray (Pam)	11 sprays (1/3 second each)	29	0.0	0
Garlic, fresh, raw	1 clove	4	1.0	1
Nutmeg, ground	1 tsp	12	1.1	0
Pimento (pimiento), canned	1 tbsp	3	0.6	2
Tabasco sauce	1 tsp	1	0.0	30
Vanilla extract, pure	1 tsp	12	0.5	0
Worcestershire sauce	1 tsp	5	1.0	65

Adapted from *Choose Your Foods: Exchange Lists for Diabetes* (American Dietetic Association and American Diabetes Association, 2008).

SECTION THREE

Put Healthy Eating into Action

Chapter 19

Change Your Eating Behaviors Slowly

What You'll Learn:

- that managing diabetes, especially eating healthfully and being physically active, is a day-to-day (and continuous) challenge
- that the best way to change your eating and activity habits and take care of your diabetes is to make changes for good, one step at a time and over time
- how to determine what behaviors to change and how to set and evaluate them
- that honesty with yourself and your health care providers is the best policy
- how keeping records can get you on and keep you on track

Managing Diabetes: A Tough Assignment

As you start to observe your current habits (yes, that's step one!) and work hard to change them, give yourself a pat on the back. Don't expect too much of yourself. Changing your behaviors and making them stick for good is hard work that requires effort and persistence. Learn to give yourself positive messages. Don't expect perfection or the impossible. You will have days when you are successful and days that just don't go as you planned.

Learn from your positive and negative experiences. Learn how to set yourself up for success and how to remove hurdles and roadblocks that are self-imposed or imposed by others. Don't let other people in your life—your family, health care providers, or coworkers—expect too much of you or set you up for failure. All you can do is the best you can do each day.

Diabetes To-Do List

- ☐ Purchase healthy foods
- ☐ Put together healthy meals and snacks
- ☐ Practice portion control with restaurant foods
- ☐ Walk 30 minutes nearly every day
- ☐ Check blood glucose a few times a day

These are just a few of the to-dos on the long list of healthy behaviors you're advised to adopt to manage your weight and your diabetes. Yes, way easier said than done! To integrate these healthy behaviors into your life is no easy task in today's fast-paced, convenience-driven world. These daily tasks are even tougher if your current eating and exercise habits don't merit a gold star for healthiness.

Making Behavior Changes

As you make behavior changes to live a healthy lifestyle, remember to take it one step at a time. Some of these goals may take months or even years to achieve. Keep the phrase, Rome wasn't built in a day, in mind! You'll have the best shot at getting to and staying at a healthy weight (remember you only need to lose a few pounds and then work at keeping them off) and keeping your ABCs on target when new healthy behaviors become your new lifelong behaviors.

The good news is that making just a few behavior changes to eat healthier and be more physically active can have a huge effect on your weight and your ABCs. This chapter gives you a process to make behavior changes slowly but surely.

Be Ready, Willing, and Able to Change

You may have people around you telling you that you have a problem with your weight or that your blood glucose is out of control, but do you think and accept that these are problems? If you don't, your efforts to make lifestyle changes aren't likely to succeed. You may even resent or be angry at the people pushing you to make changes. To succeed at changing behaviors, you need to acknowledge that **you** have a problem and then you **need** to be ready, willing, and able to change. Some experts refer to this as a readiness to change continuum.

Experts in behavior change say that to make a change, you need to accept that you have behaviors that you need to change. Also, you need to believe that changing the behaviors is important to you. In other words, there are valuable reasons for you to make the changes. For example, you want to live long enough to see your grandchildren grow up. You need to have more reasons to change

> ● **QUICK TIP**
>
> You are more likely to succeed if you break the behavior changes up into small actions. Think about a few actions you are ready, willing, and able to change now. Leave other behaviors that you don't feel ready, willing, and able to change for a later time.

your behaviors than reasons to continue your current ones. Behavior change experts also say that you must have confidence in your ability to make these behavior changes.

Choosing What to Change Now

To choose which behaviors to change first, get to know YOU and your habits better. Be honest with yourself. Learn what, where, when, and how much you eat during the day, at night, on the weekends, and so on. Think about where and when you buy food. You might want to keep food records for a few days to get a true picture of your food and eating habits (see the form on page x at the beginning of the book or use one of the many free online tracking programs or handheld device applications—see list on page 279). From your answers, you see your strengths and the areas in which you would benefit by making some changes. Answer the "Get to Know Yourself" questions in each chapter in section 2 to help you gain insight into your current food habits.

Start by choosing a few behavior changes that are easy for you to tackle and may have the biggest effect on your weight and blood glucose control. Pick one change that has to do with eating and another with physical activity. If you successfully change one habit, you're more likely to tackle the next more eagerly. For example, an easy change for you might be to eat healthier food for your nighttime snacks or to switch from whole milk to fat-free. A more difficult change would be to start eating breakfast if you never have.

When you set behavior change goals it's important to make them realistic. If your goals are too general or overly ambitious, you won't achieve them. Consider setting your goals using the SMART format. Each letter of the word SMART is an element of a realistic behavior change goal.

Here are some examples of behavior change goals. Notice that these goals are not vague like, "I will eat more fruit" or, even less specific, "I will eat healthier."

SMART Goals

Letter	Abbreviation for	Definition
S	Specific	Narrowly define your goal.
M	Measurable	Choose a frequency for the goal. How many times a day or week will you do this?
A	Attainable	Make the goal challenging but something that you can accomplish.
R	Realistic	Make the goal something you can do within the confines of your current life.
T	Time-frame specific	Limited in time frame—set short term goals that help you achieve them.

Current Behavior #1: You eat breakfast on the run from a fast-food spot or the cafeteria at work, Monday through Friday. Your usual choices are a sausage biscuit, a bagel with a thick layer of regular cream cheese, or a mega muffin and a banana.

Behavior Change Goal: For the next month (short time frame), on two days each week (measurable), I will choose one of these healthier breakfasts: a whole-wheat English muffin with jelly and a small banana or a half bagel with light or fat-free cream cheese with an orange or half grapefruit (specific and realistic).

Current Behavior #2: You realize that you consume little or no milk or yogurt over the course of a week.

Behavior Change Goal: For the next two weeks (short time frame), on three days each week (measurable), I will buy an 8-ounce carton of fat-free milk with my lunch or take a container of refrigerated non-fat sugar-free fruited yogurt to eat as an afternoon snack (specific and realistic).

Set at least one and not more than three behavior change goals at a time. Record your goals on paper or using a handheld device or online program. Keep them handy where you will see them often. If you wrote them down, post them on the refrigerator, on your bathroom or bedroom mirror, or in your purse or wallet.

Now, it's your turn. Write a few goals based on what you've learned about your eating habits.

Evaluate Your Success

The last (and repeating) lap in this behavior change cycle is to evaluate your success. Once the time period you set to practice your goal is over, look at the goals you set. Ask yourself these questions:

- Did I meet my goals?
- If not, why not?
- Were they unrealistic?
- Was the time frame too long?

If you were successful, give yourself a BIG pat on the back and a non-food reward. If you didn't reach your goals, then make your goals easier to accomplish or choose another goal that you can achieve more easily.

Your Next Step

Start the behavior change cycle again. Choose a few new goals to work on. Practicing a new behavior for two weeks or a month does not mean that this new behavior has become a lifelong behavior. It's easy to slip back to old behaviors.

Practice the new behaviors faithfully over time. It can take about six months before the new behaviors become your way of life. For instance, you always remember to stick a piece of fruit in your briefcase before you leave home in the morning and eat it during the afternoon. Maybe you automatically choose a garden salad with light dressing at a fast-food restaurant rather than French fries, or you feel sluggish if you do not get your 20-minute after-lunch walk at least three days a week.

If you use this behavior change process, before long you'll find yourself at a healthier weight, and there's also a good possibility that your ABCs will improve. Always keep in mind that you may need to start, increase, or add a medication to achieve your ABCs.

Create a Partnership with Your Provider

Your health providers now have more tools and strategies than ever before to help you manage your diabetes. These tools include new oral and injectable medications for people with type 2 diabetes, quicker-acting and longer-acting insulins for people with either type of diabetes, and medications that help manage diabetes complications. Work to find health care providers who will work with you as a partner in your diabetes care and in your efforts to change your behaviors. Don't let providers tell you what to do without your input.

Honesty Is the Best Policy

One element of a good partnership is honesty. Be honest with your provider about what you are ready, willing, and able to change. Be honest about your current lifestyle. Don't agree to make behavior changes that you know are simply impossible or agree to take a medication that doesn't fit your daily schedule.

Work in partnership with your provider to craft a diabetes care plan that works for you. Make sure you continuously review your behavior goals, your blood glucose levels, and other lab results to make sure you are hitting your target goals (see chapter 1, page 5). There's no doubt that honesty is still the best policy—for yourself and your diabetes health providers.

Record Keeping Matters

Very few people like keeping records, whether it's food, physical activity, blood glucose, or weight. It's simply time consuming and a bother; however, studies continually show that regular record keeping is one of the most important differences in helping people make and maintain behavior changes, as well as take and keep weight off. It's valuable to keep records of your blood glucose checks, the foods and amount you eat, the physical activity you do, and whatever else you and your provider feel will help you achieve your goals. Keep records the way that is best and most time efficient for you. Pen and paper is fine; however, you may want to investigate what online tools and handheld applications might make the job easier.

Online Record Keeping Tools

The computer, handheld device, and Internet have made record keeping easier. Online tracking tools are a dime a dozen—actually many are free to use, while some charge a small one-time or monthly fee.

Explore several of these websites. Many online tools interface with a nutrient database, have tools to track the calories burned with physical activity, recording blood glucose checks and more. There are also applications to download to your handheld device of choice. Some diabetes-specific sites allow you to track your blood glucose checks and when you had certain tests done. Weight loss sites, such as Weight Watchers, sparkpeople.com, or fitday.com, have even more tools. Spend a few minutes checking out the tools that might work for you.

You don't always need to record everything. Maybe you decide that for the next two months you want to see if you can make walking part of your daily diabetes care plan. You may want to track the time you walk, the length of the walk, and occasionally the walk's effect on your blood glucose. Maybe during this time you don't need to keep food records, too.

Find time to keep records. Are you an early bird? Does it make sense to record yesterday's information early the next morning? Or are you up late and have time to update your records before you retire for the night? Are you forgetful and cannot remember what you ate for longer than an hour or two? You'll probably need to record information immediately.

A Sampling of Online Resources for You

– www.fitday.com
– www.sparkpeople.com
– www.myfooddiary.com
– www.calorieking.com
– www.nutritiondata.com:
– www.diabetes.org/myfoodadvisor
– www.mypyramidtracker.gov
– www.weightwatchers.com
– www.healthengage.com

Use Your Records to Observe and Make Changes

Use your records to see whether you are successfully making the behavior changes you set for yourself or if you need to revise your goals. Use the records to understand your stumbling blocks, actions that you find helpful, and the effects of tweaks in your diabetes regimen. Bring your records when you visit your health care providers.

Talk about the blood glucose patterns you're observing. For example, you may find that your blood glucose is always higher after dinner than after lunch, or you may want to use your records to get suggestions. For example, if you find that you just can't fit in enough fruits and vegetables each day, you might like to get a few suggestions to help accomplish your goal.

Ask your health care provider whether you should be recording anything else. For instance, if you are only recording your blood glucose levels before meals, and they are always between 80 and 160, you might be surprised to find that your A1C is 8.4%. This number shows that your average blood glucose is near 200. Perhaps you should check your blood glucose 2 hours after meals to see how high it goes. Record keeping is an ongoing process. Think about what you want to learn and what changes you want to make.

Charles's Story

Charles is now officially willing to say that he has diabetes. About seven years ago, when he was 67, his doctor told him that his blood glucose was slightly elevated. His doctor prescribed a blood glucose–lowering medication to lower his blood glucose. He also encouraged Charles to stay away from sweets. At that time, Charles was 25 pounds overweight. His doctor also said it would be a good idea to take off a few pounds. Charles's doctor did not recommend that he see a dietitian or get any other education about diabetes. He did send Charles to an ophthalmologist (eye doctor) because he complained about his vision.

Charles went back to see his doctor every six months or so. A week before he went to these visits, he would stay away from sweets and take off a couple pounds by eating smaller portions. When his doctor checked his fasting blood glucose, it was never much above 160 mg/dl.

Then, two years ago, Charles began having some troublesome symptoms—feeling tired, urinating a lot, and seeing spots in his eyes. He went back to his doctor, who increased Charles's dose of one blood glucose–lowering medication and added another. The doctor also advised Charles again to limit sweets and to take off a few of his extra (now 30) pounds. This time the doctor recommended that Charles see a dietitian to help him with his weight and blood glucose levels. He also recommended that Charles go back to the ophthalmologist. The doctor suspected that Charles may have developed eye damage as a result of many years of high glucose levels.

Charles went to the eye doctor and found that he did have some vision problems because of diabetes and would need some laser surgery, which the ophthalmologist could do. The eye doctor also recommended that Charles get his ABCs into target and take his diabetes seriously.

Charles decided to go see the dietitian. He was scared about the damage that diabetes was doing to his eyes, so he was ready to be honest and to make some changes. When the dietitian asked what he usually eats—as much as he hated to do it—

(continues)

Charles's Story *(continued)*

he told the truth. He admitted that he eats sweets at least once a day and fried foods several times a week, even though he knows those foods aren't healthy for him.

Charles says he isn't much for fruits and vegetables but tries to eat one of each a day. The dietitian asked him which changes he would be willing and able to make to eat healthier. Charles set a few healthy eating goals based on his current food habits and what he is willing to do. He will try to eat at least two servings of fruit and two servings of vegetables each day. He will try to limit sweets to smaller portions four days a week and fried foods to once a week.

The dietitian talked with Charles about how important it is to be more active. Charles will start to walk for 15 minutes, three times a week. He will also keep food records during three days of each week—two weekdays and one weekend day. She gave him the links to a couple of free websites to look at their food tracking tools.

The dietitian also encouraged Charles to check his blood glucose. Charles hates doing these checks, but he agreed to do it once a day. Together, they agreed on a schedule of blood glucose checks at different times once a day to give Charles a sense of what his blood glucose is at various times during the day. The dietitian also gave him a book to record blood glucose levels, the time he does the checks, his medication, and any comments or questions he has about the blood glucose results. Charles will come back in about a month to discuss his progress with these behavior change goals.

Planning: A BIG Key to Healthy Eating

What You'll Learn:

- why planning—from meals to market to table—is a key to healthy eating
- why thinking about and gathering the foods you need on hand can save you time and money
- how to stock your pantry and refrigerator for healthy eating
- steps to take before you leave for the supermarket
- how to pick quick and easy family favorite recipes
- tips to shop smart in the supermarket aisles
- guidelines for keeping food safe in your home

Planning Is a Key to Healthy Eating

To eat healthfully day to day and week to week, you need to get into a groove that includes planning. First, spend a few minutes to plan the meals you'll prepare and eat during the next week. Then, draft your shopping list by assessing which foods you have on hand and which foods you'll need to buy. These steps may seem time consuming, but the shopping trap that many people fall into—often because of the availability of 24-hour supermarkets, convenience stores, and restaurants—costs you in three ways: health, time, and money. Check out the details below.

Health

If you grab a fast-food meal here or there, you usually end up eating fewer fruits, vegetables, and whole grains, and more high-fat meat, fat, sugars, and sodium. You may also find yourself buying food when you are most hungry and vulnerable to unhealthy choices. A key to healthy eating is to keep as much unhealthy food out of the house as possible. If foods that you have a weakness for aren't in your house, then it's much easier not to eat them. Granted, this strategy is easier for some people than it is for others, depending on the number of people in the house, their food preferences, and their willingness to change their eating habits.

> ● **QUICK TIP**
>
> A key to healthy eating is to keep as much unhealthy food out of the house as possible.

Time

If you wait to think about what you'll make for dinner until your ride home from work or other daily activities, you're more likely to opt for a convenience or fast food. If you don't have food at home, you are likely to have to purchase lunch at a cafeteria or restaurant; however, if you have foods ready at home for quick dinners—a frozen pizza with salad, an extra portion of last night's dinner, or an individual portion of leftovers that you can microwave and eat with a starch and vegetable—then you can have a healthy meal on the table in no time.

Money

If you buy food at convenience stores, eat in restaurants, order foods to go or have them delivered to your home, or cruise through fast-food drive-in windows, your money goes far more quickly than it does if you plan and shop weekly in the supermarket.

The goal is to spend a bit more time planning so that you save time when it comes to putting together healthy meals.

Time to Plan What You'll Eat

You'll need to find a few minutes to plan your meals, take stock of your pantry, refrigerator, and freezer, and develop a shopping list. Once you get in this habit, you'll find you can do it in about 15 minutes. Obviously, the amount of time it takes you depends on whether you are feeding one, two, or eight. Figure out a convenient time—perhaps early in the morning while you're sipping your morning beverage, late at night while winding down, or on a Sunday morning before your weekly supermarket run.

Is this true for you? You get into a food groove—you buy the same foods over and over week after week and then prepare and serve the same meals repeatedly. Don't consider yourself boring. This is common, and it's a good thing, because it makes your planning process much easier. Follow these steps. First, develop your food inventory and shopping list system that will work for you. You'll find an example later in this chapter. These tools can help you track the foods on your shelves, the foods you've run out of and need to replace, and the foods you'll need to buy for the next week. You may want to keep a running list on a whiteboard or piece of paper on a bulletin board in your kitchen.

You may want to take advantage of one or more of the shopping tools available on the websites noted in chapter 19 or explore other websites or handheld device apps. More people today use shopping services that receive your food order and deliver the foods to your door. There are web-based meal and menu planning programs that provide you with a shopping list of the foods you'll need. Look first at some diabetes-focused websites that help you do this. There are also online services that will deliver fresh or frozen meals to your doorstep. Though some of these services may seem costly at first, if you analyze the cost versus your time and your desire to eat healthier, one or more of these services may fit your lifestyle quite well.

Which Foods Do You Need?

Step one is to figure out which foods you'll need to have in the house to make the meals you've planned and to have the other foods you need. Start by asking yourself these questions about the next week:

- Which foods will I eat for breakfast?
- Will I eat lunch at home, bring it to work, or eat it elsewhere? If so, what do I need to buy?
- How many dinners will I eat at home? What will I make each night? Can I make a double batch of one or two recipes and freeze a few portions?
- If you want to make a certain recipe, review it to make sure you have all the necessary ingredients. Add the ingredients you're missing to your shopping list.
- Which beverages do I need to have on hand?

Let the answers to these questions help you take inventory of what you have on hand and what you need to buy. The more detailed your answers to these questions, the more complete your shopping list will be, and the more you'll decrease your need to pop into the supermarket for a few items on the way home. If one of your goals is to eat more fruit, think about when you'll eat it and which fruits you'll need to have. If your goal is to eat two servings of fruit a day, perhaps you'll try to eat one at breakfast and then bring the second one in your brown-bag lunch. If that is your plan and you shop once a week, how much fresh fruit, canned fruit, or dried fruit do you need to have on hand?

Which Foods Will You Buy?

Once you know the foods you'll need to have on hand for the next few days or week, it's time to take inventory. Check what you need against what you have in the freezer, refrigerator, and pantry. This is where a running list of what's been used up is handy. Keep your inventory list where you can immediately make notes when you are running low on something. Also, if you have the space, keep a backup supply of some staples, such as salad dressings, oil, canned broth, and frozen pizza.

Create an Inventory and Shopping List

Spend a few minutes at your computer. Think about the foods you usually buy and always want to have in your pantry. Type these in your food inventory. Divide the foods you buy into categories based on the usual floor plan of a supermarket. Start with this list. Obviously, you buy non-food items in the supermarket as well. Put them on your list. Take the list and look in your freezer, refrigerator, and pantry to check on any items you've missed putting on your inventory list. Add these in. If you want to keep a certain number on hand or make note of the size that you buy, record this information. Use it when you check your inventory to make sure you keep your stock at the level you want.

Once you have this list as a file on your computer, print out a few copies. Always keep a few inventory lists on your kitchen bulletin board. Revise your inventory list as the foods you want in the house change. Take your list to the supermarket with you and let it guide your purchases. This simple tool can greatly speed your planning as well as your shopping trips. See page 289 for a sample of the categories from the Food Inventory and Shopping List I developed and use to speed my shopping trips.

It may take some time to put these planning steps into action, but they will save you time and money.

Meal and Menu Planning

Today, people are cooking and preparing fewer meals at home. This trend is the result of our busy lifestyles and the availability of foods—whether in supermarkets, convenience stores, or restaurants. In fact, today's mammoth supermarkets have become a cross between a supermarket and a restaurant with the amount of ready-to-eat foods they sell. Although you can learn to eat healthy restaurant meals (see chapter 23 for guidance), it is easier to eat healthier at home. It's easier to serve and eat the vegetables and fruits or the whole-grain pasta or dinner rolls. It's easier to eat less sodium and less fat when you start with basic and fresh foods. And, perhaps most important, it's easier to eat smaller portions. If you've fallen into the eating out rut because you don't like to prepare meals at home, use these tips to start eating at home more often.

Think Simple

Use some of the ready-to-eat foods in the supermarket today to your advantage. They can make preparing meals at home quite easy. Try steaming precut vegetables, putting salad from a bag or box in a bowl, or dicing up rotisserie chicken (minus the skin) and placing it on a bed of salad greens. Review the chapters in section 2 to find easy ways to get the foods you need to meet your healthy eating goals. If you eat fewer restaurant meals and prepare more healthy meals at home each week, you'll soon be eating healthier.

Choose Quick-to-Fix Recipes

When you have the desire to prepare a food from a recipe, choose quick-to-fix recipes. Develop a list of five to 10 of your family's

Food Inventory and Shopping List

Dairy	Fresh Fruit	Fresh Vegetables	Breads and Starches	Cereals	Frozen Foods
Fat-free milk, 1/2 gallon	Apples (4)	Lettuce, bag	Whole-wheat sandwich	Cheerios	Pizza, cheese (2)
Yogurt, plain, quart	Bananas (3)	Lettuce, other	Raisin bread	Granola	Peas
Yogurt, fruit, 6 ounce (5)	Grapefruit	Peppers, red and green	Tortillas	Bran Flakes	Corn
Cottage cheese, 1%	Oranges (6)	Mushrooms	Pita pockets	Shredded Wheat	Fruit
Parmesan cheese	Mango	Red onion	Rice, brown	Oat bran	
Jarlsberg cheese	Blueberries	Onions	Couscous	Oatmeal	
Eggs	Kiwi	Potatoes	Pasta, whole-wheat		
Margarine, stick	Other	Cucumber	Grains		
Margarine, tub		Carrots			
Orange juice with calcium, 1/2 gallon		Tomatoes, grape			
Other		Tomatoes, whole Vegetables for week			

favorite easy recipes. Always have the ingredients on hand for three to five of these recipes. Put the ingredients you need on your food shopping and inventory list. This way, you'll always be able to come home and prepare a meal with the items you have on hand.

The following checklist provides you with helpful criteria for choosing quick-to-fix recipes. You can use the list to go through your recipes and see if any of your family's favorites fit the criteria. Use these criteria to choose new healthy recipes to add to your collection.

Common Features of Quick-to-Fix Recipes

✔ a limit of five to eight ingredients
✔ ingredients that are easy to find and easy to keep on hand
✔ easy to prepare (also include recipes that may take some time to cook but make good leftovers, like soup or stew)
✔ recipe follows the guidelines for healthy eating
✔ recipe pairs well with or contains vegetables and whole grains
✔ everyone in the family enjoys it
✔ leftovers store well
✔ recipe travels well as a brown-bag lunch

Get Ready to Shop

You have planned your meals and snacks, taken your food inventory, and created your shopping list. With your shopping list in hand, you are ready for your organized trip to the supermarket. Few people relish this trip. Supermarkets keep getting larger. There are endless aisles, food and nutrition labels to read, and ever-lengthening ingredient lists. But you have learned the steps to make the most of your trips to the market and to keep them as few and far between as possible.

Use these tactics to save you time and money:
- **Shop at the same market regularly.** Because you know where things are, you'll shop faster. Ask for help as soon as you need

it. Generally, the employees can save you time and energy looking for this or that item.

- **Shop as infrequently as you can.** Your shopping frequency depends on your family's size, the amount of fresh produce you buy, how much you can carry, and so on. The more organized you are and the more storage space you have, the less frequently you can shop.
- **Go to the market when it is not crowded.** Many markets are open 24 hours a day. Try to avoid shopping between 5 and 7 p.m.
- **Shop at one store where you can buy almost everything.**
- **Try not to shop when you are hungry.** An empty stomach means a fuller shopping cart.
- **Let your shopping list be your guide.** Try not to throw in impulse items. (It may be best to leave the kids at home if you can.)
- **Remember, the healthiest foods are usually around the perimeter**—fruits and vegetables on one wall, meats and poultry down another, and dairy foods along another wall.
- **Do not walk every aisle.** If you know you do not need items on a particular aisle, move on to the next, especially if there are aisles with foods you are better off leaving behind.
- **Read Nutrition Facts labels and ingredient lists to make sure that you know what you're buying and that the food fits into your meal plan.**
- **Find and buy the same foods week after week that satisfy your taste buds and nutrition needs.** Then you don't spend too much time reading food labels. Watch for bargains and new foods. Read the Nutrition Facts labels and see if the food is right for you. Variety is good.

Tips to Keep Your Foods Safe

The Dietary Guidelines now include keeping your food safe as an important part of staying healthy. The guidelines note that the biggest food safety problem is the spread of bacteria that cause food-borne illnesses. Two websites that offer helpful information are www.fightbac.org and www.foodsafety.gov.

The Dietary Guidelines provide the following simple recommendations to help you keep your food safe:

- Wash your hands with soap often. Be particularly careful about washing your hands when you handle raw meat, poultry, eggs, or seafood. These foods are more likely to carry problematic bacteria.
- Clean surfaces in the kitchen that come in contact with foods.
- Wash fresh fruits and vegetables—even the ones you will cook. Remove outer layers if they have them (i.e., cabbage, lettuce).
- Do not wash meat and poultry. This will help prevent the spread of bacteria.
- Separate raw, cooked, and ready-to-eat foods when you are shopping and storing foods.
- There's no need to wash ready-to-eat, pre-washed produce if you keep it properly refrigerated and use it by the date specified on the package.
- Cook foods to a safe temperature to kill microorganisms.
- Properly chill foods that need refrigeration or freezing. Make sure your refrigerator is set to about 40 degrees Fahrenheit and the freezer to about 0 degrees Fahrenheit.

Leo's Story

Leo has had type 1 diabetes half his life. He is 34 years old and works as an auto mechanic. Leo lives by himself. He takes four shots of insulin a day, tests his blood glucose regularly, and manages to keep his weight steady.

Leo has high blood pressure. He needs to limit the amount of sodium in his food. Leo's doctor has described how high blood pressure can affect Leo's eyes, kidneys, and heart. He suggested that Leo make an appointment with a dietitian. Leo and the RD discussed his diabetes care and meal planning. Leo was honest and talked about the problems with his eating plan. Leo needs to eat a lot of food—he's 6 feet 2 and very active—but the foods he chooses are not always the healthiest.

Some days Leo eats a healthy breakfast, but other days he gets a fast-food sausage biscuit or two English muffins with egg, cheese, and ham. He takes lunch to work a few days a week—several sandwiches of ham, bologna, or salami. He buys potato or corn chips and a fruit drink on the job. Two nights a week, Leo eats a frozen dinner; other nights, he has a home-cooked meal with a meat, starches, and vegetables. He orders in pizza with pepperoni and extra cheese once a week, and he eats one or two dinners out each week.

The RD focused on the high-sodium foods Leo eats. She listed the major ones—cold cuts, canned soup, convenience foods, and cheese. Foods that are low in sodium, she said, are often healthy foods like grains, fruits, and vegetables. Leo said that he shops irregularly and keeps little food in the house. That is one reason he ends up at restaurants or orders pizza. The RD suggested that Leo plan meals and snacks for the week, put together a shopping list, shop, and start the week with a full kitchen.

The RD gave Leo a few quick recipes to try—vegetable beef stew, bean and barley soup, and chicken, rice, and broccoli casserole. They talked about choosing lower-sodium foods for breakfast and lunch and using spices and dried herbs rather than the salt shaker.

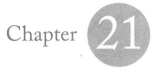
Control Your Portions

What You'll Learn:

- how portions have grown
- that controlling your portions is one of the most important tools you have to eat healthfully
- why you're likely to overeat unless you consistently weigh and measure your foods
- that weighing and measuring your foods at home will help you guesstimate portions better when you eat out
- portion control tools
- tips and tricks to eat the correct portions at home
- tips and tricks to eat the correct portions of restaurant foods

Portion Distortion

Portions of foods, whether you eat them at home or in restaurants, are often oversized. Research shows that the more food people are served, the more they will eat. Portions began to grow about 20 to 30 years ago, and so did the number of people who became overweight and obese. Portions are not the only reason people have gained weight, but they are certainly one BIG factor.

● QUICK TIP

To lose weight and to maintain your weight loss, you'll need to eat small portions of some foods, like starches, meats, fats and sweets, and put all the portion control tools and tips you learn here into practice.

People have lost sight of reasonable food portions. Have you? Reacquaint yourself with reasonable portions to eat healthier and lose weight. First, learn the servings of food you need to eat at meals and snacks by checking the serving sizes of the foods provided at the ends of the chapters in section 2.

To gain some perspective on how portions have grown, consider these comparisons in the Portion Distortion Quiz from the National Heart, Lung, and Blood Institute (www.nhlbi.nih.gov):

Food	Portion 20 Years Ago	Portion Today
Bagel	3-inch diameter, 140 calories	6-inch diameter, 350 calories
Cheeseburger	330 calories	590 calories
Spaghetti and meatballs	1 cup pasta, 3 small meatballs, 500 calories	2 cups pasta, 3 large meatballs, 1,000 calories
French fries	2 1/2 ounces, 210 calories (today's small order at a fast-food restaurant)	7 ounces, 610 calories (today's large order at a fast-food restaurant)
Turkey sandwich	1 sandwich on 2 slices bread, 320 calories	1 sandwich on large roll, 820 calories

Just a Few Calories Here and There Add Up

Losing weight and keeping it off are very difficult tasks, and accomplishing these goals can come down to a few hundred calories above your daily target day after day. Obviously, this difference of a few hundred calories can come from overeating, but it can also come from not weighing and measuring foods so that you eat proper portions. It just doesn't seem possible that an extra half cup of carrots or another teaspoon of margarine makes a big difference, but it does. It is worth noting that people commonly underestimate the amount of food and calories they eat. Some research estimates this total to be about 500 calories a day. On the flip side, people overestimate the amount of physical activity they do and the calories it burns.

You may overeat by 200, 300, or 400 calories each day. Perhaps you grab a piece of fresh fruit that is larger than the serving size, or you have an extra 1/3 cup of pasta, or an extra ounce of chicken. You might think it's okay because these foods are on your "healthy" eating plan, but extra calories here and there add up, and they can add up to enough calories to make a difference in your weight loss and blood glucose management.

Portion Control Tools

Here is a list of the portion control tools you'll want to have. Most of them you probably already have in your kitchen. A few of them may need dusting off for more frequent use.

Measuring Spoons

Make sure you have a set of measuring spoons that includes 1/2 teaspoon, 1 teaspoon, 1/2 tablespoon, and 1 tablespoon. When you use these measuring spoons, you'll see that there are 3 teaspoons in 1 tablespoon. Don't rely on the teaspoons and tablespoons from your silverware. They vary in size based on style and won't give you exact measurements.

Portion-Control Tools in the Home

Have these measuring tools handy. You may have them stored away.
Dig them out, dust them off, and find them some counter space.
Keeping them in view increases their use.

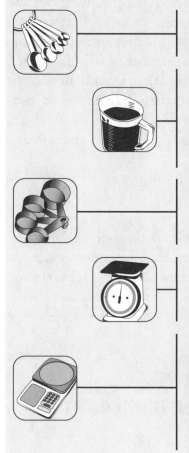

Have set of measuring spoons that includes
1/2 teaspoon, 1 teaspoon, 1/2 tablespoon,
and 1 tablespoon.

Have a 1-cup measuring cup with lines showing
1/4, 1/3, 1/2, 2/3, and 3/4 cup measures.
A liquid measuring cup should be clear (glass or
plastic). To measure liquids correctly, set the cup
down and bend down at eye level to make sure the
liquid reaches the proper line.

Have a set of measuring cups that includes 1/4-cup,
1/3-cup, 1/2-cup, and 1-cup measures. Choose the
correct size for your serving, and fill it to the top.
Level it with the flat edge of a knife.

Use an inexpensive ($5 to $15) food scale to
measure foods measured in ounces, such as fresh
fruit, bagels, potatoes, snack foods, cereals, baked
goods, meats, fish, and cheese.

More expensive scales ($25 to $190) are available. They measure more precisely in ounces,
pounds, grams, or kilograms and may provide
the gram weight and grams of carbohydrate
based on an internal database, which certainly
helps with carb counting (*www.diabetesnet.com* is
good resource for these scales).

Measuring Cup for Liquids

You'll need a 1-cup measuring cup with lines showing 1/4, 1/3, 1/2,
2/3, and 3/4 cup measures, too. A liquid measuring cup should be
clear (glass or plastic), so you can see through it. To measure liquids

correctly, set the cup down and bend down at eye level to make sure the liquid reaches the proper line.

Measuring Cup for Solids

To measure solids, get a set of measuring cups that includes 1/4-cup, 1/3-cup, 1/2-cup, and 1-cup measures. Choose the correct size for your serving—for example, of cereal or rice—and fill it to the top. Level it with the flat edge of a knife. For instance, if you want to cook 1/2 cup of uncooked hot cereal, measure it in a 1/2-cup measure and level it off to eliminate any excess.

Food Scale

Get at least an inexpensive ($5–$15) food scale. You will mainly use it to measure foods that you measure in ounces, such as fresh fruit, bagels, potatoes, snack foods, cereals, baked goods, meats, fish, and cheese.

Upscale Food Scale

More expensive scales are available, but they are not necessary. You could spend $25 to $190. On the lower priced end, the food scale measures ounces, pounds, grams, and kilograms. On the high end are digital scales that give you an exact measure instead of making you read between the lines. There are scales that actually give you the gram weight of the food and the grams of carbohydrate in that amount of the food. A good resource for these scales and other diabetes resources is www.diabetesnet.com (The Diabetes Mall).

Eyes

Don't underestimate a well-trained and honest set of eyes. Your eyes are an invaluable measuring tool because you always have them with you—even in restaurants.

Portion-Control Tools Away From Home

It is one thing to have measuring equipment at home, but like most Americans, you probably eat many meals away from home. Have no fear! When you're on the road, your eyes and hands become your portion-control tools. They work well at home, too, once you have correct portions nailed down.

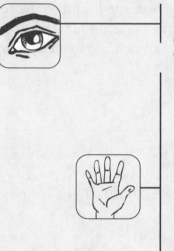

Don't underestimate a well-trained set of eyes. Your eyes are an invaluable measuring tool because they travel with you. Just make sure they are honest!

- Thumb tip (from tip of finger to first knuckle) = 1 teaspoon
- Thumb (from tip of finger to second knuckle) = 1 tablespoon
- Two fingers lengthwise = 1 ounce
- Palm of hand = 3 ounces (A regular-sized deck of cards is 3 ounces)
- Tight fist = 1/2 cup
- Loose first or cupped hand = 1 cup

Note: These guidelines hold true for most women's hands, but some men's hands are much larger. Check out the size of your hands in relation to various portions.

The Nutrition Facts on the Food Label

The Nutrition Facts label on most packaged foods today is one of your best resources because it must list the serving size. Best yet, it's free and widely available. The serving sizes on food labels today, unlike those before 1994, are regulated by the FDA. These are the serving sizes that food manufacturers must use to comply with the food-labeling law; however, they are not necessarily the same serving sizes as the servings used in this book. The servings in this book are based on those in *Choose Your Foods*, published by ADA and American Dietetic Association, 2008.

Take care not to confuse the weight in grams listed next to the serving size with the grams of carbohydrate in one serving listed next to "Total Carbohydrate." They are different. All the nutrition information on the Nutrition Facts label is based on one serving. You can use the serving sizes to help you learn what reasonable portions are. (Learn more about the Nutrition Facts label in the next chapter.)

From Raw to Cooked

How do you figure out how much raw meat, poultry, or seafood you need to prepare the right amount of cooked food? Here are some guidelines:

- Raw meat with no bone: use 4 ounces raw to get 3 ounces cooked.
- Raw meat with bone: use 5 ounces raw to get 3 ounces cooked.
- Raw poultry with skin and bone: use 4 1/4–4 1/2 ounces to get 3 ounces cooked. The extra 1/4 to 1/2 ounce accounts for the skin. (Remove the skin before or after cooking but before you eat it.)

Weigh and Measure Foods Often

Our portions are way out of line with what we need to eat. It's important that you familiarize yourself with reasonable portion sizes. The more you weigh and measure your foods and any beverages with calories, the more precise your portions will be . . . and the more successful you'll be at controlling your weight and glucose; however, it's unrealistic to try to weigh and measure every food you eat every time you eat it, so here's a realistic plan.

When you first start to follow a healthy eating plan, weigh and measure your foods as frequently as possible. Take the time to get your portions in line with the amounts you should eat. Gradually, you can weigh and measure your foods less frequently. If you think you're estimating your portions accurately, you can weigh and measure your foods

● **Q U I C K   T I P**

Keep in mind that the more often you practice weighing and measuring your foods and beverages at home, the easier it is to estimate correct servings when you eat away from home. You'll have well-trained eyes.

once a week. Perhaps you do it over the weekend when you have a bit more time or even once a month, or maybe you do well with the amounts of some foods, but you continue to overestimate others, like nuts, pasta, or meat.

Always weigh or measure new foods. Occasionally weigh or measure the foods and beverages you regularly eat to check that portions are still accurate. Quiz yourself occasionally. Serve yourself dry cereal, a serving of cooked pasta or rice, or 3 ounces of cooked meat. Then use your tools to see how close you are.

Another time to go back to weigh and measure your foods is when you see your blood glucose levels or your weight start to plateau, if you are trying to lose weight or if you are trying to maintain your weight. If you are honest with yourself, your servings will be accurate more times than not.

Tips and Tricks to Control Portions at Home

- Use your measuring tools to get and keep your eyes in line with proper portions. Always keep your measuring equipment—spoons, cups, and scale—in an easy-to-grab location. If you weigh and measure foods at home, you will have an easier time guesstimating portions when you eat out.
- Use smaller plates and bowls. Less food looks like more food on smaller plates. Dinner plates have gotten bigger and bigger. If you have a medium-sized plate, use that for dinner. You'll avoid being tempted to overfill your plate.
- Don't serve family style. Avoid putting bowls, pots, or casserole pans on the table. It makes it too easy for everyone to overeat. At least make people get up and get some exercise on their way for seconds!
- If you are used to "eating seconds," try this. Split your smaller portion in half, so you can look forward to having seconds but not overeating.
- If it's just you eating, don't leave the extras out when you sit down to eat if you don't want to eat them. Put the leftovers away before you sit down.
- When you buy produce—fruits, vegetables, and starches—buy the smallest pieces you can find. Look for small apples, bananas, and potatoes. Or buy large pieces and be prepared to eat half a piece.
- When you buy meat, fish, or poultry, buy what you need for the meal, rather than too much. This will limit overeating. If you are making hamburgers for four and want 3-ounce cooked hamburgers, then buy 16 ounces (1 pound) of meat. If you are buying smoked turkey at the deli to make four sandwiches with 2 ounces of meat, then buy as close to a half pound (8 oz) as you can. Make each sandwich with an equal amount of turkey.

Tips and Tricks to Control Portions of Restaurant Foods

- Steer clear of items with portion descriptors that are large (unless you split them). Among these are giant, grande, supreme, extra large, jumbo, double, triple, double-decker, king size, and super. Seek out portion descriptors that shout "small"—junior, single, petite, kiddie, and regular.
- Avoid all-you-can-eat restaurants or buffets. They simply encourage overeating.
- Don't fall for deals in which the "value" is to serve you more food so that you can save money. That's not a value to you. Opt for smaller amounts of tasty food.
- Be creative with the menu. Don't automatically order a main course. Opt for a soup and salad, an appetizer and soup, or a half portion. Or eat family style—share a few items with your dining partners. This is easy to do in Asian restaurants and is getting easier in other restaurants with the movement toward smaller plates or tapas.
- Split, share, and mix and match menu items to get what you want to eat in the portion you want to eat it. That's menu creativity!
- Use the fine-tuned estimating abilities that you have mastered from weighing and measuring your foods at home. Estimate what you should be eating rather than eating what they serve you. Use your eyes and those handy hand guides at your fingertips.
- If you know that the portion you'll be served will be too large, ask for a take-home container when you place your order. Put away the "second serving" before you dig in.

Sarah's Story

Sarah learned the hard way that portion control matters. Sarah first found out that her blood glucose was high at a health fair sponsored by her employer. It was 324 mg/dl. She quickly made an appointment to see her doctor to report her high blood glucose level and to see whether she really had diabetes. Indeed, her A1C was 8.3%—clearly over the 7.0% threshold to diagnose diabetes (the use of A1C to diagnose diabetes has recently been encouraged by ADA rather than using blood glucose results). Her doctor said that she clearly had diabetes. He put her on a small dose of the blood glucose–lowering medication metformin. This, he said, would bring her blood glucose out of the danger range. He felt that if Sarah could start a walking program and lose a few pounds, she would drastically improve her blood glucose level for the time being. He noted that these actions might also improve her blood lipids and her blood pressure, which were both teetering toward abnormal.

Sarah is about 35 pounds overweight, so her doctor suggested that she visit with a dietitian to develop a weight-loss plan. Sarah knew that she had some hard work ahead. She made an appointment to see a dietitian. Sarah left the dietitian's office with a healthy eating plan for between 1,200 and 1,400 calories a day. The eating plan seemed reasonable to Sarah, and it included three meals and a snack at night.

Sarah returned several weeks later and was frustrated by her lack of weight loss. She and the dietitian talked about weighing and measuring portions. Sarah said that when it came to fruits, vegetables, and starches, she depends on her eyes to judge portions. Sarah thought that a little extra here and there of these "healthy" foods would not add up to many calories. The dietitian said that those extras can make the difference, especially when you're trying to lose weight and can't spare too many calories. The dietitian showed Sarah these examples:

- an extra 1/4 cup of cooked oatmeal = 40+ calories
- a 6-ounce rather than a 4-ounce banana = 30+ calories

(continues)

Sarah's Story *(continued)*

- a 6-ounce rather than a 4-ounce apple = 30+ calories
- an extra 1/4 cup of green peas = 40+ calories
- an extra 1/2 cup of asparagus = 25+ calories
- 1 extra teaspoon of canola oil in a salad = 45+ calories

These few extras add up to 210 calories over just one day. If you add extras day after day, it can mean the difference between achieving your weight-loss and blood glucose goals or not. Sarah and the dietitian talked about the tools Sarah needs to weigh and measure her foods at home, as well as some strategies to use at the supermarket and in restaurants.

Sarah was determined to see the needle on the scale go down at her next visit to the dietitian. She dug out her measuring cups, teaspoons, and dusty old food scale. When she was in the supermarket gathering her apples, oranges, bananas, potatoes, and tomatoes for the week, she put them one by one on the food scale. Sure enough, the apples, potatoes, and bananas were several ounces larger than the target serving size. With oranges and tomatoes she was on the mark.

When Sarah wanted to eat her usual breakfast of dry cereal, rather than pouring it straight into the bowl, she took the time to pour it into the measuring cup first. She was heavy-handed with cereal. That was also true for meats—a half ounce here and an ounce there. As for fats, even though she uses the reduced-calorie versions of mayonnaise, cream cheese, and salad dressing; she was surprised when she read the Nutrition Facts to see that her servings were too big. Sarah was now convinced—control of portions is a key to healthy eating. And the best proof? When Sarah saw the dietitian a month later, she'd lost 2 pounds, and her blood glucose was closer to her target range.

Chapter 22

Lean on the Food Label

What You'll Learn:

- how the food label and the Nutrition Facts label can help you choose healthy foods and eat them in proper servings
- the information required on a food label and Nutrition Facts
- which foods must have a Nutrition Facts label
- similarities and differences in serving sizes between the food label and the diabetes serving sizes
- the meaning of nutrition claims and health claims
- tips for using the food label and the Nutrition Facts label to make healthy food choices

The Food Label—A Fountain of Facts

With today's food labels, you have more useful and accurate nutrition information at your fingertips than ever before. Although all of this information can be overwhelming, you can easily learn how to make sense of all this information and use it to help you make healthy food choices. Think of food labels, Nutrition Facts labels, and ingredient lists as your assistant in the supermarket.

Much of what you see on your food labels is required by federal laws and/or regulations implemented by the Food and Drug Administration (FDA). The Food Safety and Inspection Service of the U.S. Department of Agriculture (USDA) regulates meat and poultry products, and its regulations generally parallel the FDA's regulations. The current regulations that guide the nutrition labeling of foods were implemented in 1994. The only major change to the Nutrition Facts label since then occurred in 2006, when trans fat and information about certain food allergens began to be required by law. Small changes in the food labeling regulations are made regularly and there is currently an effort to overhaul the Nutrition Facts label, but that could take a few years. To keep abreast of food labeling information and regulations, visit www.fda.gov.

Food Label Facts

You'll find the following information on food labels:

- name of product
- weight of product
- address of the manufacturer
- ingredients used in product, listed in descending order by weight
- Nutrition Facts label with specific nutrition information per serving
- standardized nutrition claims (can only be used if certain nutrition criteria are met)
- standardized health claims (can only be used if certain nutrition criteria are met).

Foods with the Facts

Nutrition labeling is required for almost all packaged and processed foods, but there are a few exceptions: very small packages of food with no room on the label, bulk foods like cereals or nuts that are sold from barrels, foods with no nutrients, like coffee, tea, spices, and herbs, and foods produced by very small companies.

Through a voluntary point-of-purchase program, you can find the Nutrition Facts for: 20 of the most commonly eaten fresh fruits and vegetables, 45 of the best-selling cuts of fresh meat and poultry, and 20 of the most common types of fresh seafood.

A weak link in food labeling law is regulations for nutrition information for restaurant foods. The current food labeling regulations require nutrition information for restaurant foods about which health or nutrient-content claims are made on restaurant menus, signs, or placards; however, many of the large chain restaurants now provide nutrition information on their websites. Also, several cities (New York City), municipalities, and states (including California) have now passed labeling laws for restaurants with more than 20 outlets selling the same foods. Learn more about which nutrition information is and isn't available in restaurants in chapter 23.

The Fine Print of the Nutrition Facts Label

Most Nutrition Facts labels must contain at least certain key nutrition information. Some products, because of their size or the type of product, can use an abbreviated label that provides less information. Some manufacturers choose to provide you with more information or are required to do so because of one or more nutrition or health claims they make for the food. Find the Nutrition Facts label from a frozen entrée of Enchiladas with

Spanish Rice and Beans on page 312 and the explanation of each term on page 313–314.

Serving Sizes Are Your Reference

Manufacturers can't make up serving sizes for their foods. Serving sizes for nearly 150 categories of foods are standardized, and companies must use these standards. The standard servings are intended to be a typical serving, but they tend, for many people, to be on the small side. (In reality they can provide you with a sense of an amount of food you should eat!) The serving size must also be provided in household measures, such as cup or tablespoon, or it must list the number of items, so you can get a good sense of the quantity. For example, the serving size on a cracker label might read 15 crackers (28 g/1 oz). The nutrition information provided on Nutrition Facts is for one serving of most foods.

FDA Servings versus Diabetes Servings

The standard FDA-defined servings that you find used on foods may or may not be the same as the diabetes servings used in this book. You'll get to know the common diabetes servings and be able to compare them to the serving sizes on the Nutrition Facts label. The chart on page 311 gives you a few examples. You'll see that some servings are the same and some are different.

If the serving sizes are the same, then it is easy to use the Nutrition Facts as is. If they are different and you want to assess the Nutrition Facts for one serving, do some math. For example, suppose you are reading the label of regular margarine, and the serving size is 1 tablespoon. The diabetes serving size is 1 teaspoon. To get nutrient information for 1 teaspoon, you need to divide the numbers on the Nutrition Facts by 3, because there are 3 teaspoons in 1 tablespoon.

Comparison of Food Serving Sizes

Food	Food Label Serving	Diabetes Serving
Refrigerated yogurt (plain, nonfat)	1 cup	1 cup
Ice cream (light or frozen yogurt)	1/2 cup	1/2 cup
Dry cereal	30 g/oz	30 g/oz
Salad dressing (reduced-calorie)	2 Tbsp	2 Tbsp
Butter or margarine (regular stick)	1 Tbsp	1 tsp
Fruit juice	8 oz	1/3–1/2 cup
Salad dressing (regular)	2 Tbsp	1 Tbsp

Enchiladas with Spanish Rice and Beans

A —

Nutrition Facts

B — **Serving Size** 1 package (285g)

C — **Servings Per Container** 1

Amount Per Serving

D — **Calories** 330   **Calories from Fat** 50

% Daily Value* —— P

E — **Total Fat** 8 g   **12%**

F — Saturated Fat 1g   **5%**

Trans Fat 0g

G — **Cholesterol** 0 mg   **0%**

H — **Sodium** 740 mg   **31%**

I — **Total Carbohydrate** 53 g   **18%**

J — Dietary Fiber 9 g   **36%**

Sugars 4 g

K — **Protein** 9 g

L — Vitamin A 20%   •   Vitamin C 30%

Calcium 6%   •   Iron 15%

M — *Percent Daily Values are based on a 2,000 calorie diet. Your Daily Values may be higher or lower depending on your calorie needs.

	Calories:	2,000	2,500
Total Fat	Less than	65g	80g
Sat Fat	Less than	20g	25g
Cholesterol	Less than	300mg	300mg
Sodium	Less than	2,400mg	2,400mg
Total Carbohydrate		300g	375g
Dietary Fiber		25g	30g

N —

O — Calories per gram:

Fat 9   •   Carbohydrate 4   •   Protein 4

Enchiladas with Spanish Rice and Beans

Nutrition Facts Label Components

A   Title: Nutrition Facts.

B   Serving Size.

C   Servings Per Container. The nutrition information is for one serving. For example, this frozen entrée contains one serving, so the nutrition information is for the whole package.

D   Calories and the number of calories from fat in one serving.

E   Total Fat is the total number of grams of fat in one serving.

F   The two types of fat that must be listed are saturated fat and trans fat. Note that this information is indented from Total Fat and is in lighter print to indicate that these two types of fat are subcategories of Total Fat. Trans fat has been required since 2006. Manufacturers may also choose to list mono-unsaturated and polyunsaturated fat; however, if a nutrition or health claim is made, they must provide this information.

G   Cholesterol is listed in milligrams.

H   Sodium is listed in milligrams.

I   Total Carbohydrate is the total number of grams of carbohydrate in one serving.

J   The grams of two types of carbohydrates—dietary fiber and sugars—must be listed under Total Carbohydrate. Manufacturers may choose to list other sources of carbohydrate, such as insoluble or soluble fiber or sugar alcohols; this information is required if health or nutrition claims are made. (Read more about sugars and sugar alcohols in Chapter 15.) Dietary fiber and sugars are indented and are in lighter print to indicate that they are subcategories of Total Carbohydrate.

K   Protein is the grams of protein in one serving.

L   Vitamins and minerals. The percentage of the Recommended Daily Intake (RDI) in the food for two vitamins, A and C, and two minerals, calcium and iron, must be listed. If a nutrition claim is made about another vitamin or mineral, the percentage of RDI in the food for that vitamin or mineral must be on the label. For example, if a manufacturer states, "One

(continues)

Enchiladas with Spanish Rice and Beans *(continued)*

serving provides the day's need for B vitamins," the label must include nutrition information for all the B vitamins. Dry cereals often make these claims. Manufacturers can list the nutrition content for other vitamins and minerals if desired.

M   % Daily Values message.

N   The daily values are based on the amounts of each nutrient needed by a person who eats 2,000 calories a day. It's like a mini–meal plan on the label. Larger packages also must list the daily values for 2,500 calories a day. Although 2,000 calories is considered an average calorie level for adults, this level is too high for many people with diabetes who need to lose weight.

O   Calories per gram: Some of the longer labels tell you that fat has 9 calories per gram, carbohydrate has 4, and protein has 4.

P   % Daily Values for total fat, saturated fat, cholesterol, sodium, total carbohydrate, and dietary fiber are listed to the right of each nutrient. These numbers tell you what percentage of the daily value for 2,000 calories per day is in one serving of the food.

Get Personal with Your Daily Values

There are Daily Reference Values for the big nutrients that provide calories—fat, saturated fat, total carbohydrate (including fiber), and protein—and for cholesterol, sodium, and potassium, which do not contribute calories. The Daily Values on the Nutrition Facts label are based on 2,000 calories a day. This amount is considered average for all Americans, but it might be too high for you. If you eat more or fewer calories, then your personal daily values will be different from those on the label. Do the math for yourself or ask a dietitian to help you figure out your daily values. You can jot them down and carry them with you to the market to make it easier to decide whether a food fits your meal plan.

Other Items You May See on a Food Package

Ingredients: The FDA requires that ingredients be listed in descending order by weight, so the first ingredient is the one present in the greatest amount. The last ingredients are present in small amounts. Using the ingredient list along with the Nutrition Facts label can help you figure out even more about the contents of your foods.

Food Allergens: As of 2006, the FDA requires food labels to clearly state whether they contain ingredients that cause problems for people with some food allergies. Food manufacturers are required to identify, in plain English, the presence of ingredients that contain protein derived from milk, eggs, fish, crustacean shellfish, tree nuts, peanuts, wheat, or soybeans in the list of ingredients or to say "contains" followed by name of the source of the food allergen after or next to the list of ingredients. For example, if a food contains the milk-derived protein casein, the product's label will have to use the term "milk" in addition to the term "casein," so that people with milk allergies can clearly understand that there is milk in the food.

Nutrition Claim: If a nutrition claim is made on the label, the nutrition facts that justify the claim must be given. For example, if this food carried the nutrition claim "high in monounsaturated fats," then the Nutrition Facts panel would have to provide the grams of monounsaturated fat.

Put Your Daily Values into Action

When the daily value on a Nutrition Facts label is 5% or less, the food adds only a small amount of that nutrient. If the daily value is above 20%, the food provides quite a bit of that nutrient. For example, a frozen dinner provides 13% of the fat grams for the day (at 2,000 calories). If you use the rule above, 13% is a moderate amount. Consider the food and how you will use it. Is it a main course, like this frozen dinner, or is it a snack? If one serving of a snack, such as microwave popcorn, has 13% of the fat for the day, that is pretty high; however, if the food is an entrée, 13% of the fat intake is reasonable. You might want to find a lower-fat version of your snack or have a lower-fat dinner to balance the fat that you ate in the snack (See chapter 6).

Nutrition Claims Tell All

Learn to read the evidence for nutrition claims. Don't just read the bold nutrition claims without checking out the evidence that lies in the numbers on the Nutrition Facts on the label. The food labeling law requires that manufacturers give you information to support their nutrition claim. Also, only certain nutrition claims are allowed.

Since 1998, manufacturers have been able to use health claims to boast about how their foods can help you stay healthy. The process of approving health claims was put in place through nutrition labeling laws that allow manufacturers to voluntarily communicate, through the food label, about important beneficial food components that had the ability to reduce disease risk. Eight health claims were approved for use by the FDA in 1998. Since then, several manufacturers have sought and received approval for a few additional health claims. Once a health claim is approved, all manufacturers can use it.

Qualified Health Claims

Another category of health claims has been approved by the FDA, called qualified health claims. These health claims are approved with

Nutrition Claim	What the Nutrition Claim Means
Free	The product contains no amount of, or only trivial amounts of, one or more of these: fat, saturated fat, cholesterol, sodium, sugars, and calories. For example, "calorie-free" means fewer than 5 calories per serving, and "sugar-free" and "fat-free" both mean less than 0.5 grams per serving. Synonyms for "free" include "without," "no," and "zero." A synonym for fat-free milk is "skim."
Low	This term can be used on foods that you can eat often without easily exceeding the dietary guidelines. "Low" can be used for fat, saturated fat, cholesterol, sodium, and calories. These are the definitions: • low-fat: 3 grams or less per serving • low saturated fat: 1 gram or less per serving • low-sodium: 140 milligrams or less per serving • very low sodium: 35 milligrams or less per serving • low-cholesterol: 20 milligrams or less and 2 grams or less of saturated fat per serving • low-calorie: 40 calories or less per serving. Synonyms for low include "little," "few," "low source of," and "contains a small amount of."
Reduced	The product is different from the regular food and contains at least 25% less of a nutrient or of calories (e.g., reduced-fat salad dressing).
Less	The food, whether altered or not, contains 25 percent less of a nutrient or of calories than the regular food. For example, pretzels that have 25% less fat than potato chips could carry a "less" claim. "Fewer" is an acceptable synonym.

(continues)

Nutrition Claim	What the Nutrition Claim Means
Lean and Extra Lean	Used to describe the fat content of meat, poultry, seafood, and game meats. • Lean: less than 10 grams fat, 4.5 grams saturated fat, and 95 milligrams cholesterol per serving and per 100 grams. • Extra lean: less than 5 grams fat, 2 grams saturated fat, and 95 milligrams cholesterol per serving and per 100 grams.
Good and Excellent	"Good source of" means that a serving of the food provides 10–19% of the daily values for a nutrient. "Excellent source of" means that a serving of the food provides 20% or more of the daily value for a nutrient. They can also state "high in" or "rich in."
Healthy	Food manufacturers are allowed to use the term "healthy" if a food is low in fat and saturated fat, contains 600 milligrams or less sodium per serving for foods that are a meal entrée and 480 milligrams per serving for individual foods, and contains at least 10% of the daily value of vitamin A, vitamin C, calcium, iron, fiber, or protein.
More	A food that is 10% or more of the daily value when it is compared to a standard serving of the food without the added nutrients. Other terms that can be used instead of "more" are "enriched," "fortified," and "added."
Light	Light can mean two things: • A food that is nutritionally altered contains one-third fewer calories or half the fat of the regular food. If the food contains 50% or more of its calories from fat, the reduction must be 50% of the fat. • The sodium content of a low-calorie, low-fat food has been reduced by 50%. Also, "light in sodium" may be used on food in which the sodium content has been reduced by at least 50%. The term "light" still can be used to describe the texture and color of a food, as long as the label explains the intent—for example, "light brown sugar" and "light and fluffy."

"sufficient evidence" rather than the significant scientific evidence that is required for health claims. Sufficient evidence means that the scientific evidence in support of the claim outweighs the scientific evidence against the claim. A recent example of a qualified health claim granted by the FDA was for nuts: "Scientific evidence suggests but does not prove that eating 1.5 ounces per day of most nuts, such as [name of specific nut], as part of a diet low in saturated fat and cholesterol may reduce the risk of heart disease. See nutrition information for fat content." They're relatively weak statements.

Test the Nutrition Facts

Use the Nutrition Facts to see if the foods you buy or new foods you want to purchase pass your test to be a healthy food choice. Read the food label and the Nutrition Facts carefully and then answer these questions:

- Is the portion realistic for you, or will you need to count it as more than one serving?
- How many calories are in a serving?
- How many grams of fat are in a serving? What is your daily value for fat?
- Do the advertising and nutrition claims on the front match the Nutrition Facts?
- Does the food fit into your meal plan and, if so, in which food group or groups?
- Are you comfortable having this food in the house, or is it better to not have it around to help you avoid the temptation?
- If it is a convenience, ready-to-eat food that is likely to be expensive, can you make a healthier and less expensive version at home? A homemade recipe can be lower in calories, fat, and sodium. It can also contain fewer additives. For example, consider making your own hot cocoa, popcorn, soup, and pasta dishes.

Guides for the Supermarket Aisles

Gather purchasing guidelines from the list below. They will help you zero in on specific numbers on Nutrition Facts labels and shop for the healthiest foods.

Grains

- Buy your favorites and try new ones—brown rice, couscous, quinoa, barley, millet, and bulgur. Look for the most whole grains and fiber per serving.
- Buy the plain grains, not the boxed ones with seasonings.
- You can store dry grains easily for a long time, so it's no problem to keep them on hand for a quick meal.
- They contain little or no fat and are easy to prepare.

Hot Cereals

- Buy whole grains—oatmeal, oatbran, quinoa, or wheatena.
- Have a few on hand for variety.
- Look for cereals with the most fiber per serving.
- Use a combination of water and fat-free milk in cooking for more calcium.

Dry Cereals

- Buy whole-grain high-fiber cereals.
- Look for 4–5 grams of dietary fiber per serving (at least).
- Keep the sugars under 5–6 grams per serving and fat below 1–2 grams.

Pasta and Noodles

- Buy the dry kind; they are the least expensive, and they store the longest.
- Purchase the whole-wheat or whole-grain variety for extra fiber and other nutrients.

Breads, Bagels, and Rolls

- Go for whole-wheat or whole-grain varieties.
- Get at least 2–3 grams of dietary fiber per serving.
- Cut the fat by limiting biscuits, croissants, doughnuts, and higher fat specialty breads, such as prepared garlic or focaccia bread.

Crackers

- Buy fat-free and reduced-fat types, but be sure they really are.
- Keep fat to 1–2 grams per serving.
- Buy whole-grain varieties to get 1–2 grams of dietary fiber per serving.

Starchy Snack Foods

- Go for naturally fat-free and whole-grain pretzels and baked tortilla chips.
- Purchase light, fat-free, and reduced-fat varieties, but make sure they are what they say.

Beans

- Have several types of dried beans on hand. They store well.
- Stock a few types of canned beans. They are quick to prepare.
- They have zero fat, plenty of soluble fiber, and loads of other nutrients.
- Buy fat-free varieties of refried beans, baked beans, and vegetarian chili.

Starchy Vegetables

- Have potatoes on hand to cook in the microwave—whole or chopped.

- Try red (new) potatoes or Yukon gold potatoes for a small, sweet, tasty variety.
- Buy fresh sweet potatoes and winter squashes; they stay fresh for a couple weeks and are packed with vitamins and minerals.
- Keep frozen corn and peas around. Sprinkle them on salads or in soups or use them as a healthy starch serving.

Vegetables

- Eat fresh or frozen vegetables often.
- Keep canned or frozen ones in your kitchen, so you'll always have vegetables on hand.
- Avoid frozen vegetables packed with high-fat sauces and seasonings.
- Keep individual cans of vegetable juice on hand for a quick gulp of vegetables.

Fruits

- Eat fresh, whole pieces of fruit often.
- Keep canned or frozen (no-sugar-added) fruit in your kitchen, so you'll always have fruit on hand.
- Buy canned or frozen, no-sugar-added fruit or fruit packed in its own juice.
- When you buy fruit juice, make sure you look for 100% fruit juice.
- Avoid fruit drinks and fruit-flavored carbonated drinks with a lot of calories.

Milk and Yogurt

- Look for nonfat and fat-free products.
- For yogurt, choose nonfat, sugar-free; fat-free, sugar free; or nonfat (higher sugars content).
- Choose calcium-fortified milk if you can find it.

Red Meats—Beef, Lamb, Pork, and Veal

- Choose the leaner cuts as often as possible.
- Go for lean or extra-lean ground meat.
- Buy lean or extra-lean cold cuts and hot dogs.
- Think about the portions you want to serve when you purchase the meats.

Poultry

- The skinless breast with no wing is lowest in fat.
- Try turkey parts.
- Buy ground turkey or low-fat turkey sausage to replace ground meat in recipes. Check the label; ground turkey with the skin included is higher in fat.
- Usually a whole bird is cheapest and boneless breast is most expensive per pound.

Seafood

- Keep canned tuna (water-packed), salmon, crabmeat, clams, or imitation crabmeat on hand for a quick meal.
- Buy any type of fresh or frozen fish unbreaded.
- Choose the higher-fat fish—salmon, mackerel, or bluefish—to up your intake of omega-3 fats.

Cheese

- Go for cheeses with less than 5 grams of fat per ounce—light, part-skim, and reduced-calorie.
- Cottage cheese—buy 1%, nonfat, or fat-free.

Fats

- Oil: Stock one healthy all-purpose oil, such as canola or sunflower oil. (You might try a blend of soy and canola oils that is very low in saturated fat.) Also keep olive oil around if you enjoy the taste in salad dressings and in cooking.

- Margarine and spreads: Use a light tub variety (about 5 grams of fat per tablespoon). Try to get one that has zero trans fats.
- Mayonnaise: Use low-fat or reduced-calorie (about 5 grams of fat per tablespoon) mayonnaise.
- Salad dressing: Reduced-calorie dressing has about 5 grams of fat per 2 tablespoons; fat-free has less than 20–30 calories per 2 tablespoons. Best yet, make your own with a healthy oil.
- Sour cream and cream cheese: Use light or fat-free types, as long as you enjoy the taste.

Cookies and Cakes

- Only buy them if you can control the portions you eat.
- Try to buy ones that are trans fat free.

Frozen Desserts

- Buy light and fat-free varieties, but remember that they are not calorie-free.
- Keep calories in the 100–150 range per 1/2-cup serving.

Free Foods

- Keep plenty of fat-free items in the pantry, such as herbs, spices, sauces, and seasonings.
- These add flavor to low-fat meals.

Soups

- Keep cans or dry packages for quick meals or snacks. Look for the reduced or low-sodium types.
- Buy broth-based or bean-based soups and limit the creamy varieties. Opt for lower-sodium versions.

- Dry packages work well as a traveling meal or snack.
- Dry packages of vegetable, onion, or other soups can double as dip mix. Make sure you watch the sodium content.

Frozen Entrées

- Buy reduced-calorie or low-fat varieties to limit fat and keep serving sizes under control.
- Keep fat down to about 3 grams per 100 grams of food.
- Keep sodium down to 600–800 milligrams per entrée.

Pizza

- Keep frozen cheese pizza on hand, and top it with fresh vegetables.
- Choose a whole-grain pizza crust.
- Purchase a pizza crust, pita bread, or bagel, and add your own tomato sauce, part-skim cheese, and vegetables.

Patricia's Story

Patricia is 54 and has had type 2 diabetes for about 2 years. She has been struggling to lose 15–20 pounds, which her doctor says will help her lower her blood glucose and improve her blood fats. Her goal is 165 pounds, and she is 5 feet, 7 inches tall. She also has problems with regularity. Her doctor suggested that foods with lots of dietary fiber would help her constipation and may improve her blood fats. Patricia had not met with a dietitian until some members of a diabetes support group said that a few visits with a dietitian had helped them.

The dietitian and Patricia talked about weight loss, blood glucose records, blood fats, and problems with constipation. The dietitian asked Patricia about the foods she buys in the supermarket and whether she understands and uses the Nutrition Facts on the food label. They found that Patricia was not eating certain foods because she was trying to make sure that no food contained more than 30% of calories from fat. They figured Patricia's daily value for fat is about 60 grams, based on about 1,800 calories each day. They looked at a few food labels, and Patricia learned how to add up the total grams of fat. She also learned to compute the calories from fat and how that adds to her total calories. She now realizes that she can enjoy reduced-calorie salad dressing, mayonnaise, and light sour cream in the proper servings as long as her total fat intake is around 50–60 grams per day or 25–30% of her total calories.

Patricia and the dietitian also looked at ways she could increase dietary fiber to help ease constipation and improve her blood fats. They determined that her daily value for dietary fiber is 21 grams. The dietitian suggested that Patricia try to sprinkle peas, garbanzo beans, kidney beans, or bulgur wheat on salads. She can also buy dry cereals that have at least 5–6 grams of fiber per serving and whole-grain breads with at least 3 grams of dietary fiber. The dietitian suggested that Patricia try to increase her fruits and vegetables to eat five to six servings each day. Patricia agreed to chart her progress and come back in a month.

Chapter

Skills and Strategies for Healthy Restaurant Eating

What You'll Learn:

- reasons it can be difficult to eat healthfully in a restaurant
- skills and strategies for eating healthier restaurant meals
- how to put together healthier restaurant meals to fit your healthy eating plan
- the healthier choices to order in a variety of restaurants

Restaurant Meals

A half century ago, eating a meal in a restaurant was a rarity. Thirty years ago it was reserved for special occasions—Mother's Day, a birthday, an anniversary. Today, restaurant eating has become a way of life in America. On average, Americans eat four meals out each week. Interestingly, about one-quarter of these meals are eaten at fast-food restaurants.

Don't feel that having diabetes prevents you from eating and enjoying restaurant meals; however, restaurant foods have some pitfalls, and you will need to arm yourself with a few critical skills and strategies to eat restaurant foods healthfully.

If you eat out as frequently as average Americans, every meal can't qualify as a special occasion, yet you may still have a special occasion mentality when you eat restaurant meals. You may think it's fine to eat larger portions, splurge on a dessert, or have a higher-fat side dish or entrée. If you eat several restaurant meals each week, you cannot continue to view restaurant meals as special occasions and stay on track with your diabetes nutrition goals. More important, this attitude can affect your goal to lose weight.

Getting to Know Yourself

If you want to change your habits about how often you eat restaurant meals, the types of restaurants you eat in, and the foods you eat there, it's worth taking a few minutes to ask yourself these questions to learn what you're doing before you can take steps toward changing any habits. Start by responding to these questions:

When do I eat out?

- Think about an average day, week, or month. Estimate the number of meals and snacks you eat away from home. Do not forget meals and snacks that you purchase at restaurants and eat somewhere else.
- Compare how often you eat out on weekdays and weekends.

*Which meals and snacks do I eat away from home
during an average day, week, or month?*

- Breakfast, lunch, dinner
- Morning, afternoon, evening/bedtime snacks

Why do I eat restaurant meals?

- Restaurant meals are convenient.
- I do not like to cook.
- I want to have someone serve me.
- I enjoy various ethnic flavors that I cannot create in my kitchen.
- I need a place and way to get together with friends, family, or business associates.
- I want to relax during lunch or at dinner after a long day.

What types of restaurants do I choose?

- Fast-food (hamburger, chicken, or seafood chains)
- Pizza or sub shops
- American fare—family restaurant, steak house, upscale continental cuisine
- Ethnic fare (fast-food)
- Ethnic fare (table service)
- Sweets, desserts, ice cream

*Which foods do I eat in the restaurants listed above
and in what amounts?*

- Write down what you usually order in the restaurants you go to (including beverages).
- Observe the foods you eat at different types of restaurants.
- How do the servings compare with the servings in my meal plan?
- Are there food groups missing from restaurant meals that should be part of my meal plan?

Do I drink alcoholic beverages when I eat in restaurants?

- If yes, how many alcoholic drinks do I have when I eat out?
- What alcoholic beverages do I usually drink?
- What is the calorie content of these alcoholic beverages?

Challenges to Healthful Restaurant Eating

There are four main challenges to eating healthy in restaurants. Learn about these. Then gather and master the skills and strategies for healthier restaurant eating.

1. **Restaurant foods can be high in fat and high in calories.** By now you know that fat makes food taste good. Restaurants love to use oils or shortening to fry; butter and cream to create sauces; salad dressing on salad; sour cream on baked potatoes; cheese or cheese sauce on sandwiches; and butter, cream, and eggs to make desserts.

2. **Restaurant foods can be high in sodium.** The high-sodium content comes from salt; ingredients like soy sauce, meat tenderizers, broth, ham, or bacon; sauces and gravies; use of prepared canned food such as soups and vegetables; and salad dressings. If you need to limit sodium and you eat out a lot, you may have to eat out less often. When you do eat out, limit high-sodium foods just as you do in the supermarket. Asian cuisines—Japanese, Chinese, and Thai—can be quite high in sodium.

3. **Restaurant meals can be high in protein (meat, poultry, or seafood).** This is particularly true in American-style restaurants—steak houses, delicatessens, sandwich shops, and family restaurants. Think of a delicatessen sandwich stuffed with 6–8 ounces of corned beef, pastrami, or smoked turkey. You know from the details of this book that this amount of meat is enough meat for two or three sandwiches.

4. **Restaurant portions can be way too large.** In America, the theory goes that more food equals greater value. Americans get taken in by this message. Unfortunately, it often encourages overeating. Not taking advantage of these deals takes some rethinking.

Skills and Strategies Galore

Use these skills and strategies to rethink the way you approach restaurant meals and to gather tips and tactics to apply when you try to eat healthier restaurant meals.

Have a Can-Do Attitude

If you believe that all restaurant meals are special occasions, even though they happen several times a week, it's time for you to perform a mental mind shift. You'll need to learn how to eat and enjoy a healthy restaurant meal without going overboard with portions or high-fat and high-sodium foods. You'll need to learn to sit back and relish other aspects of restaurant meals, like not having to wash the dishes!

Select a Restaurant with Care

Today, you can go into most restaurants and order a healthy meal if you choose. Most menus offer at least some healthier items, or you can be creative with the menu and design a healthy meal. There are restaurants where eating a healthy meal is nearly impossible, but don't set yourself up for defeat; select restaurants that offer you at least a few healthy options.

Have a Game Plan

When you cross the threshold of a restaurant, have in mind what you will order. It's likely that you've been to this restaurant many times and know the menu quite well. Don't let the menu tempt you and take you off track.

Be a Knowledgeable Fat Detective

You know that restaurant foods load on the fat. It is easy to keep a lid on fats if you learn

- the foods that are high in fats and calories, such as butter, cream, mayonnaise, sour cream, salad dressing, cheese, sausage, nuts, and avocado

- the cooking methods described on the menu that add fat, such as fried, deep-fried, battered and fried, golden brown, sautéed in butter, and served in a cream sauce
- the names of high-fat dishes, such as chimichangas (Mexican), fettuccini Alfredo (Italian), and sweet and sour whatever (Chinese).

Hold the Line on Sodium

Once you can spot the high-sodium offenders, steer clear or cut down on them and make a few reasonable special requests. Chapter 8, on salt and sodium, provides you with some tips to reduce sodium when you eat out.

Use Menu Descriptions

They can help you find healthier options. Look for foods such as broth-based tomato sauce, foods that come with lettuce and tomato, fat-free or low-calorie salad dressing, or fresh fruit. Some foods are naturally low in fat and calories, such as vegetables, pasta, dried beans, herbs, and spices. Look for healthier cooking methods (described on the menu), such as marinated, poached, grilled, blackened, served in a light wine sauce, or topped with sautéed garden vegetables. Look for dishes that have healthier ingredients, such as fajitas (a Mexican dish served with guacamole and sour cream, which you can request held or on the side), Yu Hsiang chicken (Chinese), and pasta primavera (be careful that the sauce does not have cream added).

Be Creative with Menus

Do not feel that you have to order an entrée if the portions seem huge. If restaurants want to serve too much food, then order from the appetizers, soups, salads, and side dishes. Mix and match items to get the amount of food you need to eat.

Split Menu Items

Because servings are so large, there is often enough for two. (You might need to order an extra side dish.) For example, one person orders an 8-ounce (raw weight) sirloin steak, a baked potato, and a trip to the salad bar. The other person orders an extra baked potato and a trip to the salad bar. Split the steak. Then it is just the right size, about 3 ounces cooked meat for each person. You can read many more portion control tips for restaurant eating in chapter 20.

Some good news for "splitters" is that, in many ethnic restaurants, family-style service is customary. The entire dish can be placed in the middle of the table to share. You decide how large your serving will be. Order fewer dishes than the number of people dining, or split with yourself. Order a menu item with a take-home container. When your order arrives, put half away to take home or to the office for another meal.

Share Menu Items

Share two or more menu items (depending on the number of dining partners) that complement each other and achieve the goals of your healthy eating plan. This technique outsmarts the large protein servings. For example, in an Italian restaurant, one dining partner orders chicken cacciatore, which probably has about 6–8 ounces of chicken. The other partner orders pasta with a light tomato sauce, marinara, or Bolognese. When you split the two dishes, each person ends up with 3–4 ounces of chicken and 1–1 1/2 cups of pasta. Order your own dinner salad for more vegetables, and order the dressing on the side.

Order Foods the Way You Need Them

Special requests help you trim the fat and calories. It's OK to make reasonable requests, but don't ask or expect to have a menu item re-created in the kitchen. For example, do not request that a dish like Chicken Kiev be grilled. That's simply not how it's prepared. Move on to a healthier item such as grilled teriyaki chicken or stir-fry chicken with garden vegetables served over linguine. Here are some reasonable special requests:

- Please bring my salad dressing, butter, or sour cream on the side.
- Please remove from the table or do not bring any bread and butter, chips and salsa, or Chinese noodles.
- Can the chef grill or broil this meat (poultry or seafood) rather than fry it?
- Please hold the sour cream, guacamole, shredded cheese, or olives.
- Please split this entrée into two servings in the kitchen, or bring us an extra plate.
- Can you serve this ham or turkey sandwich on whole-wheat bread rather than on a croissant?
- Can you hold the mayonnaise and bring me mustard?

Let Your Eating Plan Be Your Guide

Visualize a couple of restaurant meals. The first consists of a fast-food quarter-pound hamburger, French fries, a side salad with Thousand Island dressing, and a regular soda. The second is a Mexican meal with a basket of chips and salsa, a combo plate with one chicken taco and one beef enchilada, Mexican rice, refried beans, and a dessert of custard flan. Both of these meals paint the common picture of restaurant meals: heavy on fats, meats, and sweets and light on milk, vegetables, and whole grains. Fruit is nowhere to be seen. As you know by now, these meals are in stark contrast to healthy eating.

For starters, let your eating plan be your guide. Until you have your eating plan committed to memory, keep a copy in your wallet as a handy reference. Look at the menu and consider your eating plan.

See how you can work in whole grains. For example, are you in a Chinese restaurant that offers brown rice as an option instead of white rice? Are you eating breakfast out and can opt for whole-grain pancakes? In a sub shop, get more vegetables by asking them to load on the lettuce, tomatoes, and onions and lighten up on the fat by leaving off the mayonnaise and oil. To fit in fruit, you'll often need to bring it with you and eat it when you are back in your car or as a snack later. These are examples of how to apply the skills and strategies of healthy restaurant eating.

To help you further understand how to let your eating plan be your guide with restaurant meals and how to apply the skills and strategies of healthy restaurant eating, here are some sample healthy restaurant meals based on the actual nutrition information from the restaurant chains. These meals show you how you can closely match the number of servings from the various calorie eating plans to an array of restaurant meals. Note that the sodium content of several of these meals is high. A challenge with restaurant eating is the sodium content. See page 341 at the end of this chapter to learn where to find nutrition information for the popular chain restaurants.

Healthier Restaurant Meals

Lunch at Subway
(based on 1,200–1,400
  calories a day)
Total Servings: 3 Starch,
  2 Vegetable, 2 Meat, 1 Fruit

6" Roast Beef Sandwich on
  Honey Oat Bread (highest
  in fiber) (hold the oil, go light
  on the mayonnaise, and
  request plenty of lettuce,
  tomatoes, and onions)
Veggie Delite Salad
Italian Dressing, Fat-free
Fruit Roll-up

Nutrition Facts

Calories 470	**Calories from Fat** 135

Total Fat 15 g
  Saturated Fat 2 g
  Trans Fat 0 g
Cholesterol 63 mg
Sodium 1,425 mg
Total Carbohydrate 76 g
Protein 23 g

(continues)

Healthier Restaurant Meals *(continued)*

Dinner at Fazoli's Italian Restaurant
(based on 1,200–1,400 calories a day)
Total Servings: 3 Starch, 1 Vegetable, 2 Meat, 3 Fat

Minestrone Soup
Tuscan Chicken Bake (split in half)
Garden Salad
Dressing (request olive oil and vinegar; use 1 tsp oil and unlimited vinegar)

Nutrition Facts

Calories 490	**Calories from Fat** 198

Total Fat 22 g
    Saturated Fat 7 g
    Trans Fat 0 g
Cholesterol 63 mg
Sodium 1,890 mg
Total Carbohydrate 49 g
Protein 26 g

Breakfast at Au Bon Pain
(based on 1,400–1,600 calories a day)
Total Servings: 3 Starch, 1 Fruit, 1 Milk

Raisin Bran Muffin (split in half)
Banana (split in half)
Cafe Au Lait with Fat-Free Milk (small)

Nutrition Facts

Calories 385	**Calories from Fat** 90

Total Fat 10 g
    Saturated Fat 1 g
Cholesterol 17 mg
Sodium 515 mg
Total Carbohydrate 74 g
Protein 12 g

Dinner at Chipotle's Mexican Restaurant
(based on 1,400–1,600 calories a day)
Total Servings: 3 Starch, 1 Vegetable, 4 Meat, 3 Fat

6" flour tortillas (2)
Carnitas (pork) (1 serving)
Fajita Vegetables (1 serving)
Black Beans (split in half)

Nutrition Facts

Calories 618	Calories from Fat 243

Total Fat 27 g

Saturated Fat 6 g

Cholesterol 66 mg

Sodium 2,272 mg

Total Carbohydrate 53 g

Protein 40 g

Lunch at Pizza Hut
(based on 1,900–2,300 calories a day)
Total Servings: 5 Starch, 2 Vegetable, 3 Meat, 4 Fat

Thin 'n' Crispy Veggie Lover's Pizza (4 slices from large pizza)

Nutrition Facts

Calories 720	Calories from Fat 252

Total Fat 28 g

Saturated Fat 12 g

Cholesterol 60 mg

Sodium 1,800 mg

Total Carbohydrate 84 g

Protein 28 g

Dinner at Boston Market
(based on 1,900–2,300 calories a day)
Total Servings: 4 Starch (corn and butternut squash are starchy vegetables), 5 Meat, 1 Fruit

1/4 White Meat Chicken (no skin, no wing)
Sweet Corn (1 serving)
Mashed potatoes without gravy (1 serving)
Hot Cinnamon Apples (split in half)

Nutrition Facts

Calories 625	Calories from Fat 108

Total Fat 12 g

Saturated Fat 5 g

Cholesterol 105 mg

Sodium 1,232 mg

Total Carbohydrate 80 g

Protein 40 g

Healthier Restaurant Offerings by Cuisine

These two side-by-side lists show you some of the healthier and not-so-healthy offerings at a variety of types of restaurants, from fast-food to Chinese. As you look at these lists, think about what you typically order in this type of restaurant. Then think about how you can make a few changes to eat healthier offerings.

FAST-FOOD HAMBURGER CHAINS

Healthier Choices
Hamburger, cheeseburger, single
Grilled chicken sandwich
Grilled chicken salad
Baked potato, with chili or broccoli
French fries, small or share larger
Garden and side salads
Salad dressings, use light or use less
Chef salad (light dressing)
Roast beef sandwich
Frozen yogurt

Not-So-Healthy Choices
Hamburger, cheeseburger, double, triple, deluxe
Fried fish sandwich
Baked potato with cheese sauce

ROTISSERIE-CHICKEN CHAINS

Healthier Choices
White or dark meat (remove the skin), rotisserie, BBQ, grilled
Ham or Turkey
Chicken soup

Side Dishes
Apples and cinnamon
Corn bread or muffin
Baked beans
Corn
Fruit salad

Not-So-Healthy Choices
Dark meat, with skin
Chicken, fried
Chicken pie

Side Dishes
Caesar salad with dressing
Coleslaw
Creamed spinach or corn
Macaroni and cheese
Pasta salad
Stuffing

Healthier Restaurant Offerings by Cuisine *(continued)*

Green beans
Potatoes, mashed, pieces, baked
Rice
Steamed vegetables
Zucchini in tomato sauce

Meat sandwiches with cheese sauce
Chicken salad sandwiches

MEXICAN RESTAURANTS

Healthier Choices
Black bean, tortilla soup, or gazpacho
Mexican or taco salad
Arroz con pollo (chicken and rice)
Burritos
Enchiladas
Fajitas
Soft tacos

Not-So-Healthy Choices
Chili con queso
Flautas
Nachos or super nachos
Tacos (hard shell)
Chimichangas

Side Dishes
Black beans
Mexican rice
Pico de gallo
Hot sauces, all

Note: To eat less fat, ask for cheese, sour cream, or guacamole on the side. Request extra salsa to add flavor.

CHINESE RESTAURANTS

Healthier Choices
Wonton, egg drop, or hot and sour soup
Steamed Peking dumpling
Teriyaki beef or chicken
Chop suey or chow mein

Not-So-Healthy Choices
Egg or spring roll
Jumbo shrimp
Meat and nut dishes
Deep-fried dishes
General Tso's chicken

(continues)

Healthier Restaurant Offerings by Cuisine *(continued)*

Moo shi chicken, etc.
Shrimp with tomato sauce
Vegetarian stir-fry dishes

Sweet and sour shrimp, chicken, pork, etc.
Peking duck
Spareribs

ITALIAN RESTAURANTS

Healthier Choices
Italian bread (hold the butter)
Marinated vegetable salad
Minestrone soup
Shrimp cocktail
Pasta with tomato sauce, marinara, Bolognese, meatballs, red or white clam sauce
Chicken or veal with cacciatore, light wine, or light tomato sauce
Chicken or shrimp primavera (no cream in the sauce)

Not-So-Healthy Choices
Garlic bread or rolls
Fried mozzarella cheese sticks
Caesar salad with dressing
Cannelloni, lasagna
Pasta with pesto
Sausage and peppers
Pasta with cream and cheese sauces, Alfredo, carbonara
Chicken or veal parmigiana

PIZZA AND SUBMARINE SHOPS

Healthier Choices
Cheese pizza with vegetables
Submarine sandwiches with turkey, ham, roast beef, cheese (hold the oil and mayonnaise, and add vegetables)

Not-So-Healthy Choices
Cheese pizza with sausage, pepperoni, and/or extra cheese
Submarine sandwiches with tuna, chicken, or seafood salad; Italian cold cuts

AMERICAN RESTAURANTS

Healthier Choices
Broth-based soup
Chili
Peel and eat shrimp
Salad with light or fat-free salad dressing (on the side)

Not-So-Healthy Choices
New England clam chowder
French onion soup

Healthier Restaurant Offerings by Cuisine *(continued)*

AMERICAN RESTAURANTS

Healthier Choices

Salad with grilled tuna or chicken

Baked potato topped with chili

Fajitas

Stir-fry chicken with vegetables

Teriyaki chicken breast

Not-So-Healthy Choices

Buffalo wings

Potato skins

Tuna melt

Philadelphia cheese steak

Quiche

Ribs, beef or pork

Nutrition Information from Restaurants— Where and How?

If you frequently eat restaurant meals, you will want to learn more about the nutritional content of the foods you eat. It's best to look for exact nutrition information for these foods from these restaurants. You're in luck when you look for information from large chain restaurants that serve fast-food fare: burgers, chicken, pizza, breakfast foods, and sandwiches. Many of these large chain restaurants provide nutrition information on their websites. Search for the restaurant's website, and go to the menu information. This usually leads you to nutrition information. Unfortunately, much less information is available from the "sit down and order" restaurants—both national chains as well as independent ethnic and American restaurants.

A book published by the American Diabetes Association that you may find helpful is the *Guide to Healthy Restaurant Eating*, 4th edition, 2009. This guide provides the basics about today's diabetes nutrition and meal planning goals and strategies for healthy restaurant eating. It contains a wealth of nutrition information, including carbohydrate, calories, fat, percentage of calories from fat, saturated fat, cholesterol, sodium, fiber, and protein, along with servings or exchanges for nearly 5,000 menu items from more than 60 major restaurant chains across America.

Jeremy's Story

Jeremy had his blood glucose checked at a health fair. It was higher than normal, and he decided to get it checked by his doctor. Rather than checking his blood glucose his doctor checked his A1C level. The result was 6.8%, which showed he is at high risk for diabetes (≥ 6.5 or $\leq 7.0\%$ is high risk for diabetes).

Jeremy was relieved to hear his doctor say that, with a small amount of weight loss and walking, he may be able to prevent or at least delay the onset of type 2 diabetes for a while. Jeremy's doctor also told him that he has several other characteristics that are common in pre-diabetes and type 2. They are being overweight, having high blood pressure, and having high triglycerides. Jeremy is 45 years old and is about 35 pounds overweight. His weight has steadily crept up over the last ten years. His doctor suggested that Jeremy make an appointment with a dietitian and start to make some lifestyle and behavior changes to improve all these health problems.

Jeremy went to see a dietitian several weeks later. The dietitian asked Jeremy to paint her a picture of how he eats day to day. Jeremy said that he is divorced and lives alone. He is busy at work and with other activities in his life, so he eats most of his meals away from home. He noted that breakfast during the week might be a muffin or a bagel with a large fancy coffee drink with sugar and cream. On the weekends, he usually eats a bigger breakfast with eggs and sausage or bacon. Lunch is often a full size sub sandwich with tuna fish or Italian meats and a bag of chips. Dinner can vary even more. Sometimes Jeremy stops at a local rotisserie chicken restaurant, where he gets half a white meat chicken, a spinach soufflé, and mashed potatoes with gravy. Other nights, he might eat Mexican food or order Chinese food or pizza to be delivered.

The dietitian talked with Jeremy about eating breakfast at home a few days a week. He said he was willing to start to buy whole-grain cereal and eat a bowl with fat-free milk and a piece

(continues)

of fruit. They talked about healthier breakfast options for weekday and weekend breakfasts. For lunch, the dietitian suggested that Jeremy order a 6-inch sub sandwich rather than the large size and that he order lower-fat fillings such as turkey, ham, or roast beef. She recommended that he leave off the mayonnaise and oil and use no-fat mustard instead. Instead of chips, the dietitian suggested pretzels or, better yet, a garden salad drizzled with a lower fat salad dressing, since Jeremy eats so few vegetables. The dietitian encouraged Jeremy to bring along and eat a piece of fruit in the afternoon. They went on to discuss changes Jeremy could make with his dinnertime menus.

Jeremy was grateful that the dietitian didn't talk to him about following an unrealistic diet or encourage him to cut out all his restaurant meals. He was positive about being able to make some of the changes she suggested, and he was willing to try them out because he was motivated to stay healthy. Jeremy made an appointment to see the dietitian again in one month to check on his progress and set some additional goals.

Chapter 24

Get the Support You Need

What You'll Learn:

- why it's important to keep learning about diabetes
- how to find a diabetes educator and/or diabetes education program
- how to figure out which diabetes care expenses are covered by your health plan
- how to go local or global for diabetes support

Healthy Eating: A Key to Diabetes Care

The effect of a healthy eating plan may be greatest when you are first diagnosed with pre-diabetes or type 2 diabetes. At this early point, healthy eating matched with regular physical activity can help you lose a few pounds. That may be all you need at the moment to bring your ABC numbers into your target ranges. Over time, as your pre-diabetes may become type 2 diabetes or your type 2 diabetes now requires one or more blood glucose–lowering medications, research shows that following a healthy eating plan day to day will help you better manage and achieve your ABC goals in addition to taking the medications you need.

Most people diagnosed with type 2 diabetes will need to begin taking blood glucose–lowering medication immediately or soon after their diabetes diagnosis. It is becoming clearer that though losing a few pounds is important, it is very hard to keep them off over the years. Realize that weight loss or no weight loss, healthier eating will always help you achieve your ABC goals more easily and may help you require less medication over time.

Get the Know-How You Need to Succeed

Learning to eat healthier to get and stay healthy with pre-diabetes or diabetes takes time. You've learned a lot from your first reading of this book. Now put it on your shelf and come back to it frequently when you have questions, need suggestions or encouragement, or are ready to make more changes in your lifestyle. To increase your knowledge further, you can read other American Diabetes Association resources and take advantage of many online resources at www.diabetes.org. Because new research findings in nutrition and diabetes come out all the time and diabetes care continues to evolve, it's important to keep reading.

Get the Support You Need to Succeed

It's also important for you to get the support you need. Learning about healthy eating with diabetes is one thing, but making the all-important lifestyle changes for good is much harder. Research shows that to be successful long term, people need to stay connected. The good news is that with technology today, it's easier and more cost-effective than ever.

Be kind to yourself; remember that new lifestyle changes come slowly, but they do stick as long as you take a can-do attitude. Tackle easy habits first, and reward yourself for your successes.

Where to Get Knowledge and Support

Seek out a diabetes education program staffed by diabetes educators or find a registered dietitian who has expertise in diabetes care. Having these people as resources for knowledge and support can be invaluable to you as you strive to care for your diabetes and stay healthy for the long run. These providers can be your coaches and part of your all-important cheerleading squad. Today, and in the future, some of these services will be available online.

Find a Diabetes Education Program or Educators

Everyone with diabetes should receive diabetes education. It's vital when you are first diagnosed with diabetes and important throughout your life. There are several ways of finding the experts who can provide this education and support:

- **The American Diabetes Association (ADA):** The ADA approves diabetes education programs through an application and recognition process. Going to an ADA "Recognized Program" ensures that you receive quality diabetes education. Most often, a registered dietitian (RD) is one of the staff members of the program. The RD is also likely to be a certified diabetes educator (CDE). ADA programs are available throughout the U.S., and they usually offer diabetes education classes as well as one-to-one counseling. The services you are eligible to receive will depend on what your health plan covers or you decide to pay for. The people who provide the education are usually nurses and dietitians. Some programs may also have exercise physiologists, pharmacists, or behavioral counselors on staff. To find these ADA diabetes education programs in your area, call the ADA at 1-800-DIABETES (1-800-342-2383) and ask for the program nearest you. Or visit http://professional.diabetes.org/erp_zip_search.aspx, to find a recognized education program in your area.

- **The American Association of Diabetes Educators (AADE):** Many diabetes educators belong to this professional organization. Diabetes educators may be nurses, nurse practitioners, dietitians, exercise physiologists, pharmacists, social workers, behavioral counselors, or psychologists. Diabetes educators may provide their services in hospitals, out-patient clinics, managed-care organizations, in endocrinologists' offices, in large-group physician practices, at their own independent facilities or via online services. You will find diabetes educators at ADA-recognized diabetes education programs (see above) or in programs that have been accredited by AADE. To find an AADE accredited program, go to www.diabeteseducator.org/ProfessionalResources/accred/programs.html. You can also find a diabetes educator in your area by going to www.diabetes-educator.org/DiabetesEducation/Find.html and click on the state in which you want to find an educator. Or call the AADE at 1-800-TEAMUP4 (1-800-832-6874).
- **The American Dietetic Association:** To find a registered dietitian in your area, go to www.eatright.org, click on "Find a Nutrition Professional," and follow the instructions.
- **The Yellow Pages:** You might find a diabetes education program or registered dietitians at your local hospital, or these resources may be listed in the yellow pages. Look up "Endocrinologist" under "Physicians" in the yellow pages. Call and ask about diabetes education programs or diabetes educators who are dietitians in your area.
- **Other People:** Talk to people who have diabetes or people in a diabetes support group to see if they can recommend an education program or educators.

Health Plan Coverage and Reimbursement for Diabetes and Nutrition Education

Does my health insurance plan cover and reimburse for diabetes education (also called training) and nutrition counseling (also called medical nutrition therapy)? This question often comes up. Unfortunately, there's no simple answer for all health plans—from Medicare and Medicaid, to private health insurance plans. The answer depends on your health coverage and the state or federal regulations that apply to this plan. Today, many people who have health insurance can get coverage and reimbursement for diabetes education. You might hear this service referred to as diabetes self-management training (DSMT). You can also often get coverage and reimbursement for medical nutrition therapy (MNT).

Coverage has improved greatly over the last decade for two reasons. The first is that federal law now requires Medicare to cover both DSMT and MNT for people diagnosed with diabetes. (Note: Unfortunately, if you have pre-diabetes, these much-needed services continue not to be covered, though there is movement toward including pre-diabetes.)

The second reason that coverage of diabetes care has improved is that most states have enacted laws requiring health plans to cover these services. You can check ADA's website at www.diabetes. org/living-with-diabetes/ treatment-and-care/health-insurance-options/health-insurance-in-your-state to see if your state has such a law and to get a few details about the law.

The best way to find out what is covered is to contact a diabetes education program or diabetes

● **QUICK TIP**

To learn more about what Medicare covers (both training and supplies), go to www.Medicare.gov or call your local Medicare office. You can also find information about Medicare and coverage of diabetes supplies and education on the ADA website at www. diabetes.org/living-with-diabetes/treatment-and-care/health-insurance-options/65-and-older/medicare.html.

educator. Give them the name of your health plan, and they may be able to tell you whether their services are covered and to what degree. You can also get details about coverage from your health plan by calling the toll-free number on your health plan card or by using the plan's website. Ask which services and how many visits are covered, whether you have to go to a particular person or program, and whether you need a referral for the service from your diabetes care provider. If you feel you should be covered for DSMT and/or MNT but your health plan is denying this coverage, then ask questions and demand answers. Plead your case!

If your health plan isn't willing to cover diabetes self-management training or medical nutrition therapy or you have no health insurance, then you'll have to decide whether to reach into your pocket and pay for these services. You will probably come to realize it is money well spent. All things considered, a few sessions with a knowledgeable diabetes educator is not that expensive when compared to medications, hospitalizations, or even the cost of a restaurant meal.

Finding a Local Diabetes Support Group

A local diabetes support group can be an invaluable resource for you as you work toward your healthy eating goals. Here's how to find a local group:

- Call 1-800-DIABETES (1-800-342-2383). Find out the focus of the support group, the age range of the members, and when and where they meet.
- Call a local diabetes education program or a diabetes educator.
- Ask your pharmacist.
- Call the office of a local endocrinologist or diabetologist.
- Call a nearby hospital to see whether their diabetes program runs support groups.

Finding Global Diabetes Knowledge and Support

The Internet has given rise to many online diabetes resources, from information from national and international organizations, to government agencies and well respected health and diabetes resources. In addition, there's been a huge expansion of independent websites, blogs, social media venues, and more to help support your diabetes care efforts. Make sure that whatever resources and support vehicles you access offer trusted information.

Here are links to numerous resources and/or supportive networks, which can keep you informed and support your mission to take care of your diabetes. Consider these trustworthy sources, but always view information with a questioning eye. Reality is there's way more information than anyone can possibly digest.

Think about why and how you'll use these vehicles. Do you want to receive a regular e-newsletter, get a blog feed, connect with other people with your type of diabetes?

National and International Organizations and U.S. Government Agencies

– www.diabetes.org (American Diabetes Association) (access to e-newsletters, information, food and nutrient information, message boards and much more)
– www.niddk.nih.gov (The National Institutes of Health's institute which deals with diabetes, National Diabetes and Digestive and Kidney Diseases) National Diabetes Education Program (NDEP)
– www.ndep.nih.gov (The National Diabetes Education Program run by NIDDK)
– www.nhlbi.nih.gov (The National Institutes of Health's institute which deals with heart and blood vessel diseases and often works with NIDDK on research and programs)
– www.cdc.gov/diabetes (The Centers for Disease Control and Prevention's diabetes division known as the Division of Diabetes Translation)
– www.jdrf.org (The Juvenile Diabetes Research Foundation, a resource for research and information about type 1 diabetes)
– www.idf.org (The International Diabetes Federation, an international organization)

Diabetes Information Websites/Blogs (non organization or government affiliated)

Blogs may be independent of a diabetes information website or be within a website:

– www.childrenwithdiabetes.com (Children With Diabetes, an organization dedicated to helping children and their parents deal with diabetes.)

– www.diabetesmine.com (written by a person with diabetes about what's happening in the world of diabetes)

– www.behavioraldiabetes.org (Behavioral Diabetes Institute, an organization developed to tackle the unmet psychological needs of people with diabetes)

– www.dlife.com (dLife.com is an active website for the diabetes community, they also host a weekly (Sundays) TV show on CNBC called dLifeTV)

– www.diabeticconnect.com (a place to connect and find support from others with diabetes)

– www.diabetesdaily.com (a place for diabetes news and support)

– www.diabeticlivingonline.com (the website of Better Homes and Gardens magazine Diabetic Living filled with information and recipes)

– www.diabetesselfmanagement.com (the website for Diabetes Self-Management magazine)

– www.diabetesstories.com (the blog of author Riva Greenberg, a person with diabetes)

– www.diabetessisters.org/ (a website/blog run by a woman with diabetes for women with diabetes)

– www.tudiabetes.com (a website with many blogs run by Manny Hernandes, a man with diabetes)

– www.diatribe.us/home.php (an e-newsletter with diabetes research and product news)

Good luck on your road to healthy eating and becoming more physically active! By eating healthfully and being physically active day after day, you'll improve your chances of hitting your ABC targets—blood glucose and A1C, blood lipids, and blood pressure. When you keep your numbers on target over many years, you vastly increase your chances of staying healthy and living a long life!

Index

Other Titles from the American Diabetes Association

Complete Guide to Diabetes, 4th Edition

by American Diabetes Association
Have all the tips and information on diabetes that you need close at hand. The world's largest collection of diabetes self-care tips, techniques, and tricks for solving diabetes-related problems is back in its fourth edition, and it's bigger and better than ever before.
Order no. 4809-04; New low price $19.95

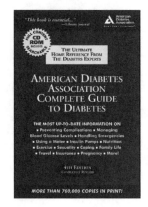

Real-Life Guide to Diabetes

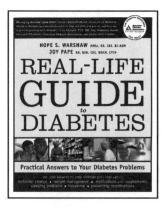

by Hope S. Warshaw, MMSc, RD, CDE, BC-ADM, and Joy Pape, RN, BSC, CDE, WOCN, CFCN
Real-Life Guide puts everything you need to know about diabetes into a one-of-a-kind book packed with the information you won't find anywhere else. Learn to prevent long-term complications, understand health insurance, work physical activity into your daily life, and control your blood glucose, cholesterol, and blood pressure.
Order no. 4893-01; Price $19.95

50 Things You Need to Know about Diabetes

by Kathleen Stanley, CDE, CN, RD, LD, MSEd, BC-ADM
Cut through the confusion, jargon, and conflicting information about diabetes care and get the simple advice you need about eating right, exercising, and staying healthy. Learn how to interpret A1C and eAG numbers, keep your love life happy, and avoid depression and burnout. Make your life easier—and a lot healthier!
Order no. 4884-01; Price $17.95

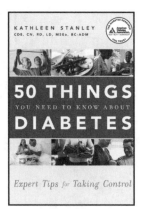